THE GREEN DYNAMO

Developing Your Athletic Skills in The Vegan Kitchen

Artem Zhdanov

Copyright

©[2024],[Artem Zhdanov]

Disclaimer

This is a fictional work. Names, characters, places, and incidents are either made up by the author or used fictitiously. Any resemblance to actual people, alive or dead, business establishments, events, or locales is entirely coincidental.

The author and publisher have no control over, and accept no responsibility for, third-party websites or content mentioned in this book. The inclusion of any website links does not necessitate a recommendation or endorsement of the views expressed within them.

While the author has made every effort to provide accurate and up-to-date information, readers should verify facts and seek professional advice before making any decisions based on the material in this book. The author and publisher expressly disclaim any duty for any adverse effects or consequences arising from the use of the information presented in this book.

About the Author

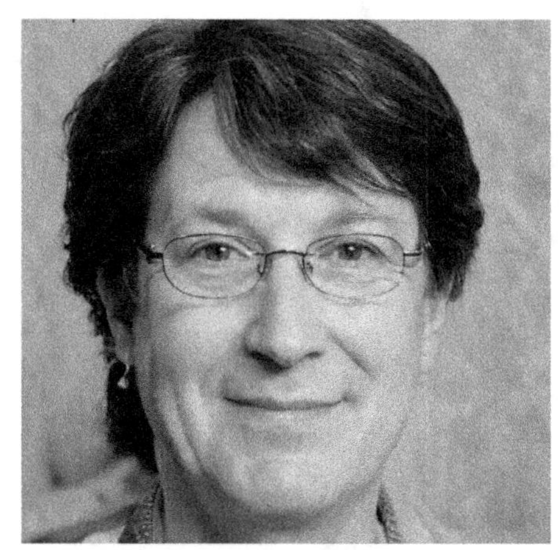

Meet Artem Zhdanov, the inspiration behind the enlightening material about vegan athleticism. Artem is a fervent supporter of plant-powered living and contributes a plethora of expertise and firsthand experience.

Artem's pursuit of the best possible health and athletic performance led him to explore the world of veganism. His commitment to investigating the relationship between fitness, compassion, and diet has established him as a reliable source among the active vegan athlete community.

Artem, who has experience in publishing, blends his knowledge with a sincere desire to impart useful advice and cutting-edge methods for plant-based diet. His meticulously designed content inspires, informs, and lifts, demonstrating his devotion to empowering people on their vegan athlete path.

Come along with Artem on this life-changing journey where he invites you to maximize your athletic potential while embracing the holistic advantages of a vegan lifestyle.

Table of Contents

INTRODUCTION   **8**
Welcome to the Vegan Athlete Lifestyle   8
Why Vegan Diets Are Better for Athletic Performance   8

Chapter 1: Nutrition Fundamentals for Vegan Athletes   **12**
Understanding Macronutrients: Protein, Carbohydrates, and Fats   12
Micronutrients: Essential Minerals and Vitamins for Peak Function   14
Tips for Hydration for Vegetarian Sportsmen   16

Chapter 2: Building a Strong Foundation   **20**
Powerhouses of Plant-Based Proteins   20
Crucial Amino Acids for the Repair of Muscle   36
High-Voltage Sources of Carbohydrates   39

Chapter 3: Power-Packed Breakfasts   **42**
Energizing Smoothie Bowls   42
Protein-Rich Waffles and Pancakes   44
Variations of Overnight Oats   47

Chapter 4: Nourishing Lunches   **50**
Lentil and Quinoa Power Bowls   50
Vegan Sandwiches and Wraps   52
Plant-Based Proteins Boost Salads' Vitality   55

Chapter 5: Satisfying Dinners   **60**
Vegan Pasta Recipes with Protein   60
Filling Bean and Grain Stews   63
Stir-Fries as Easy and Packed with Nutrients   66

Chapter 6: Snacks and Energy Boosters   **70**
Make Your Own Energy Bars   70
Nut mixtures with Roasted Chickpeas   73
Ideas for Fresh Fruit Snacking   75

Chapter 7: Recovery Smoothies and Drinks   **80**
Smoothies with Protein After Exercise   80
Electrolyte drinks that hydrate   82
Superfood Elixirs in Green   85

Chapter 8: Meal Planning and Prep Tips   **90**
7-day vegan meal plans for athletes   90
Techniques for Freezing and Batch Cooking for Busy Vegan Athletes   97
Savvy Grocery Purchasing for Foods High in Nutrients   100

Chapter 9: Vegan Supplements for Athletes   **104**
Recognizing Nutrient Shortfalls in a Vegan Diet for Athletes   104
Essential Vegan Supplements for Optimal Sports Results   107

Chapter 10: Success Stories   **112**

CONCLUSION 114
REVIEW PAGE 116

INTRODUCTION

Welcome to the Vegan Athlete Lifestyle

Set off on an adventure that goes beyond the confines of conventional sports nutrition. This cookbook serves as your entry card into a world where plant-based performance is the main attraction. This guide is designed for everyone, from seasoned athletes trying to improve their performance to beginners inquisitive about the advantages of a vegan diet.

We'll look at the combination of colorful flavors, nutrient-dense foods, and renewable energy sources in the pages that follow. The Vegan Athlete Lifestyle is a comprehensive approach to nourishing your body, mind, and soul—it's not just a diet. Prepare to be amazed by the abundance of meals that will stimulate your palate as well as improve your physical performance.

As you per use these pages, keep in mind that adopting a vegan lifestyle is all about plenty rather than sacrifice. An abundance of vitality, health, and delectable meals that will transform the concept of what it takes to be a successful athlete. Put on your equipment, lace on your running shoes, and let's explore the amazing world of plant-powered living. Time to Get Powered Up and Succeed!

Why Vegan Diets Are Better for Athletic Performance

In the quest for athletic greatness, each decision we make counts. Every choice we make, from our training program to the nutrition we feed our bodies, affects how well we perform as a whole. There's a question: Why adopt a vegan diet to improve your athletic performance?

A Harmony of Elements: A vegan diet provides an abundance of nutrients that come straight from the soil. Foods derived from plants are rich in vitamins, minerals, and antioxidants, offering a wide range of nutrients that promote proper body function. Learn how this nutrient-dense orchestra strengthens your immune system, encourages endurance, and improves healing.

Plant-Driven Healing: Discover: The science of plant-based recuperation and how it helps to reduce inflammation and speed up the regeneration of damaged muscles. Learn how antioxidants and plant proteins work together to speed up recovery so you can recover from workouts faster and return stronger.

Resilient Energy: Explore the idea of renewable energy produced by plants. The constant flow of energy from plant-based sources powers your exercises and aids in maintaining endurance during training sessions and competitions, in contrast to the peaks and crashes that are frequently linked with processed foods.

Environmental and Ethical Considerations: Explore the ethical and environmental implications of adopting a vegan diet in addition to its personal advantages. Discover how utilizing plant-based energy complies with environmental sustainability and animal welfare standards, making your journey not only a personal victory but also an investment in a healthier Earth.

Statements from Vegetarian Sportsmen: Hear the accounts of vegan athletes who have changed to a plant-powered diet and saw improvements in their performance. These testimonies offer first hand proof of the beneficial effects of a vegan diet on sports performance, ranging from higher energy levels to improved recuperate.

Handling Frequently Asked:

Questions: Talk about typical questions and misunderstandings about vegan diets for athletes. Gain the knowledge necessary to confidently follow a vegan lifestyle without sacrificing your performance or wellbeing, from protein consumption to nutrient adequacy.

You will learn the powerful reasons why a vegan diet can revolutionize your athletic path as we go through the chapters in this book. It's important to fuel your body properly for a lifetime of continuous energy, enhanced recuperation, and unmatched performance. It's not just about what you eat. Greetings from a new plant-powered athletic success.

Handling Frequently Asked:

Chapter 1: Nutrition Fundamentals for Vegan Athletes

Understanding Macronutrients: Protein, Carbohydrates, and Fats

Macrofructs are major players in the complex dance of sports performance. These three fundamental components of nutrition—protein, carbs, and fats—have an impact on everything from muscle growth to long-term energy. Let's explore the intricacies of macronutrients and learn how their interactions might enhance your vegan athletic lifestyle.

Protein: The Essential Components for Effectiveness

Explore the world of plant-based protein sources, which are the building blocks of growing and repairing muscles. Discover the differences between complete and incomplete proteins and discover how to prepare meals high in protein that satisfy your needs as an athlete. Learn the truth about plant proteins, which might be your strong partners when trying to gain muscle and stamina.

Carbs: The Energy Source for the Trip

The body uses carbohydrates as its main energy source, and for the vegan athlete, this means that maintaining endurance requires consuming carbohydrates. Discover a range of plant-based carbs, from simple to complex, and learn how to add them to your meals before and after your workouts. Learn how to carb-load for optimal performance.

Fats: The Silent Champions

Contrary to popular belief, fats are not toxic. They are necessary for the synthesis of hormones, the health of joints, and general well being. Explore the world of plant-based healthy fats and discover how to get the ideal balance for your needs. Learn about the delicious ways that fats can improve your athletic journey, from avocados to almonds.

Macronutrient Ratios in Vegetarian Sportsmen

Recognize the optimal macronutrient ratios to meet the special requirements of athletes who follow a vegan diet. Adjust your macronutrient consumption to support your unique athletic objectives, whether your concentration is on strength training, endurance, or a combination of the two. Discover the keys to longer-lasting energy and improved recuperation with careful food planning.

Schedule and Allocation

It matters not just what you eat, but also when you eat it. Examine the significance of timing your pre-and post-workout meals to get the right nutrients. To keep your energy stable and promote recovery, learn how to divide up your macronutrients throughout the day so that you're always prepared for your next workout.

Recipes that Highlight the Harmony of Macronutrients

Use the recipes in this collection to put your newly acquired knowledge into practice by creating the ideal macronutrient balance. Learn how to prepare delectable meals that can satisfy your cravings and support your fitness objectives, from protein-rich power bowls to energy-boosting snacks.

You will learn skills and acquire the information necessary to become an expert at nourishing your body for optimal performance as we explore the complexities of macronutrients. It's time to realize the benefits of a diet rich in protein, carbs, and fats and to fully realize the potential of your vegan athlete lifestyle.

Micronutrients: Essential Minerals and Vitamins for Peak Function

Micronutrients are the unsung heroes of athletic achievement, coordinating your body's many functions into a harmonious whole. These vital vitamins and minerals are important for maintaining immune system health as well as energy metabolism. Come along as we explore the realm of micronutrients and learn how to improve your vegan athletic lifestyle.

The Arsenal of Micronutrients

Take a tour through the vital vitamins and minerals that are necessary for optimal athletic function. Discover the functions that various micronutrients—from iron to zinc, magnesium to vitamin B12—play in preserving health, avoiding shortages, and maximizing your body's capacity for optimal function.

Plant-Powered Sources of Micronutrients

Explore a wide variety of plant-based foods that are high in the micronutrients your body needs. Discover how to put together a varied, nutrient-dense meal that will support your general health and athletic aspirations with anything from colorful fruits to leafy greens.

Sunshine and vitamin D

Explore the connection between vitamin D and sunshine and learn how it supports immune system function, bone health, and general vigor. Knowing how to keep vitamin D levels at their ideal levels becomes essential for long-term health and performance for vegan athletes.

The Oxygen-Carrying Iron

Examine in-depth the significance of iron for athletes, as it is essential for energy metabolism and oxygen delivery. Discover the benefits of consuming enough iron from plant sources and how iron and vitamin C work together to improve absorption in Antioxidants: Nature's Defense

Discover the world of antioxidants and how they can help prevent oxidative stress brought on by strenuous exercise. Discover the plant-based sources of vitamins, minerals, and selenium that can shield your cells from harm and promote quick healing.

Managing the Intake of Micronutrients: Recognize the delicate balance needed to provide the micronutrients your body requires. Discover how to customize your vegan diet to include a range of foods that satisfy all your needs and ensure that you have the story of micronutrients needed for long-term athletic success.

Micronutrients and Recuperation: Examine the relationship between recovery from a workout and micronutrients. Learn how these little powerhouses ensure that you recover from each training session stronger by boosting muscle repair and lowering inflammation.

You will learn more about the role that micronutrients play in your overall athletic performance as we explore the complex world of these components. It's time to upgrade your vegan lifestyle by utilizing vitamins and minerals to propel your workouts and whole path to peak performance and wellness.

Tips for Hydration for Vegetarian Sportsmen

Staying hydrated is crucial when aiming for optimal performance. If you're a vegan athlete, maintaining proper hydration involves more than just topping off on fluids—you also need to make sure your body is getting the plant-based energy it needs to function. Come discuss hydration tactics catered to the special requirements of vegan athletes.

The Value of Staying Hydrated

Recognize the reasons why maintaining proper hydration is essential to athletic performance. Learn about the physiological processes that depend on adequate hydration and how it affects your performance in your chosen sport, from temperature control to nutrient delivery.

Water: The Vital Elixir

Examine the importance of water for vegan athletes as their main source of hydration. Find out how much water you actually need depending on your body weight, degree of exercise, and surrounding circumstances. Learn the advantages of maintaining proper hydration and how dehydration affects athletic performance.

Electrolytes Powered by Plants

Explore the world of alternative plant-based electrolyte alternatives to traditional sports drinks. Learn how nature offers a variety of electrolytes to support normal muscle function, avoid cramping, and improve overall sports endurance, from watermelon to coconut water.

Foods That Will Hydrate Athletes

Examine the double advantages of eating foods that are high in water content and high into help you stay hydrated. Discover a range of plant-based solutions that will keep you hydrated and nourished during your training sessions, from delicious fruits to hydrating veggies.

Herbal Teas and Rehydrating Drinks

With tasty herbal infusions and hydration elixirs, you can up your hydration game. Discover how to make cool beverages that not only satisfy your thirst but also offer additional health advantages for vegan athletes by combining the freshness of herbs, fruits, and spices in delicious recipes.

Hydration Rituals for Before and After Exercise

Recognize the significance of drinking enough water before and after your workout. To maximize performance and effectively recuperate from training sessions, understand how to strategically hydrate prior to exercise. Learn the techniques for keeping your balance fluidly as you progress as an athlete.

Challenges with Hydration for Vegan Athletes

Discuss the common hydration issues that vegan athletes encounter, such as increased fiber consumption and possible electrolyte imbalances. Prepare yourself with workable answers to these problems and make sure your hydration plan works in harmony with your plant-based lifestyle.

Beyond Water: Vital Hydration

Staying hydrated is a way of life, not just something you do during exercise. Discover the benefits of regular hydration for your general health as a vegan athlete. Learn about the comprehensive advantages of making drinking water a priority in all facets of your life, from better digestion to increased cognitive performance.

As you go through this chapter, you will acquire a thorough understanding of hydration tactics designed with the vegan athlete in mind. It's time to hydrate for a lifetime of sustained energy, vitality, and athletic excellence—not just for your upcoming session.

Chapter 2: Building a Strong Foundation

Powerhouses of Plant-Based Proteins

Plant-based protein is the foundation of strength, endurance, and recuperation in the world of vegan athletics. Come along as we explore the vast and varied realm of plant-based protein sources, revealing the nutritional treasures that will catapult you to new heights in your sports career.

Lentils

The best plant-based protein source is lentils. It is high in protein, which is necessary for the development of our muscles and general body mass. If you are a vegetarian or vegan, they are a great substitute for animal-based proteins in your diet. Lentils also have a high fiber content, which aids in a healthy digestive system and prolongs feelings of fullness. So, adding lentils to our diets could be a terrific way to maintain our health and get the essential protein that our bodies need.

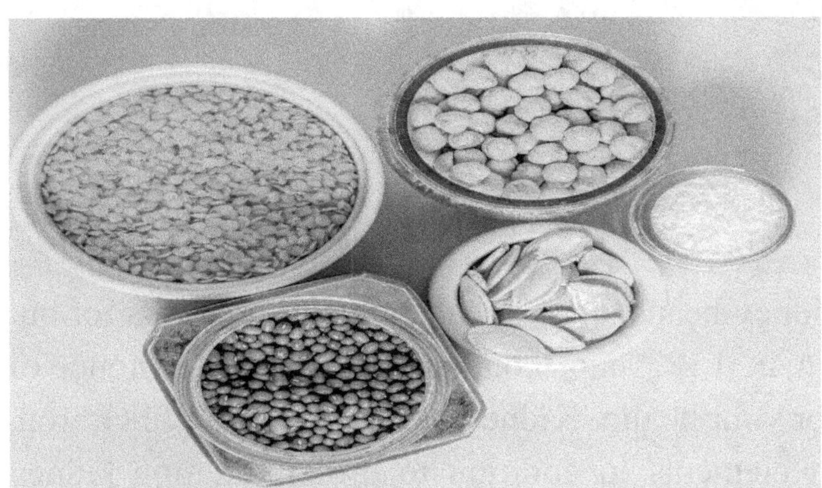

Chickpeas

One of the best vegetarian protein sources is chickpeas. Known as garbanzo beans, these little legumes are a great source of beneficial minerals. They are high in protein, which is essential for maintaining overall health and gaining muscle. The US Department of Agriculture (USDA) estimates that a serving size of 1/2 cup of chickpeas has around 7.5 grams of protein. In addition, chickpeas are an excellent source of healthy fats, iron, phosphorus, fiber, and folate. Chickpeas can be enjoyed in a variety of ways, such as as the main component in a delectable Indian stew or roasted for a crunchy snack.

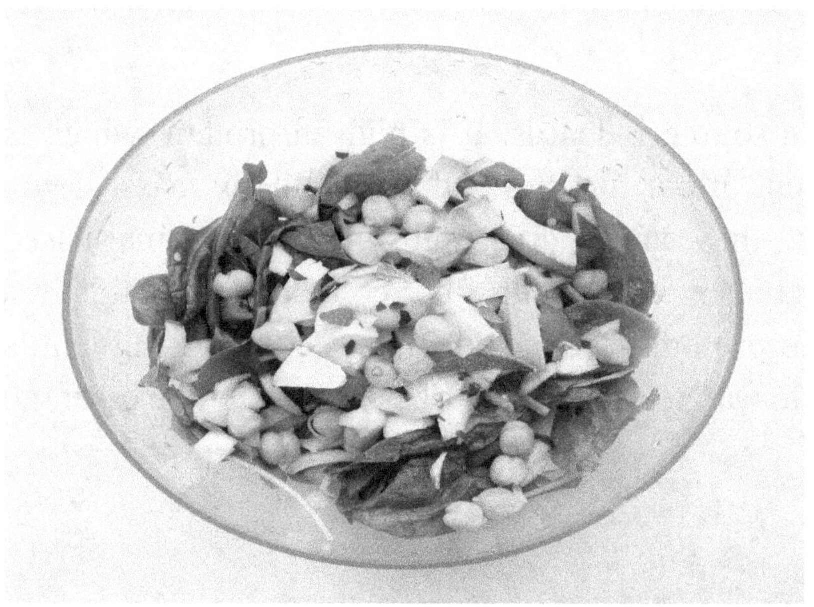

Kidney beans

Rajma, another name for kidney beans, are a great source of nutrients for our bodies. Kidney beans, even in 1 / 2 cup, contain a substantial amount of protein that may be good for your health. Kidney beans are rich in fiber, iron, folate, and other important elements in addition to protein. Eating kidney beans can help control blood pressure, blood sugar, and cholesterol levels. It's a high-protein vegetarian dish that can help you lose weight. They go well with salads, soups, and vegetarian Indian curries.

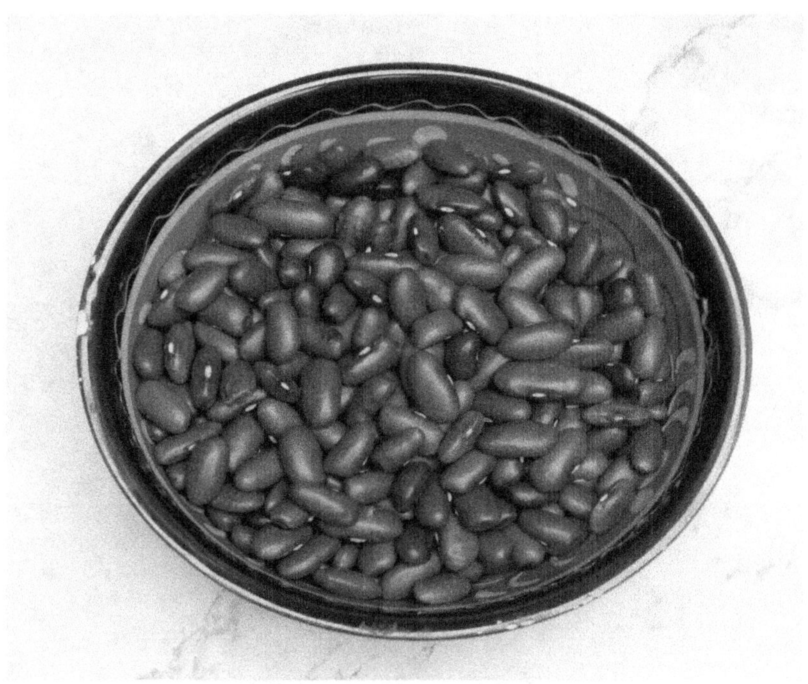

Green peas

With more than nine grams of protein in each cooked cup, green peas are a great source of protein. As a matter of fact, green peas have somewhat higher protein content than a cup of dairy milk. Green peas are rich in important elements and a good source of protein for vegetarian diets. One serving of green peas provides more than 25% of your daily requirements for fiber, thiamine, folate, manganese, and vitamins A, C, and K. They also provide good levels of iron, magnesium, zinc, phosphorus, copper, and numerous B vitamins. For vegetarians, this makes peas the first source of protein.

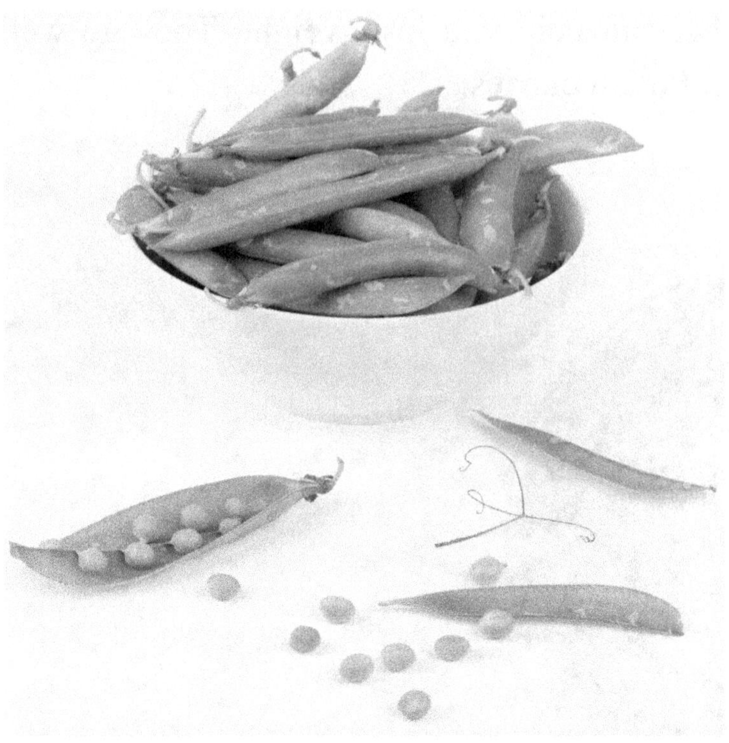

Soybeans

Among the nutritious foods that are high in protein for vegetarians are soybeans. Other vital nutrients including fiber, iron, calcium, and vitamins are also found in soybeans. The daily consumption of two to four servings of soy-based meals can yield numerous health advantages. Thus, feel free to add soy protein as a healthy food to your diet if you're a vegetarian who loves to eat a lot of protein.

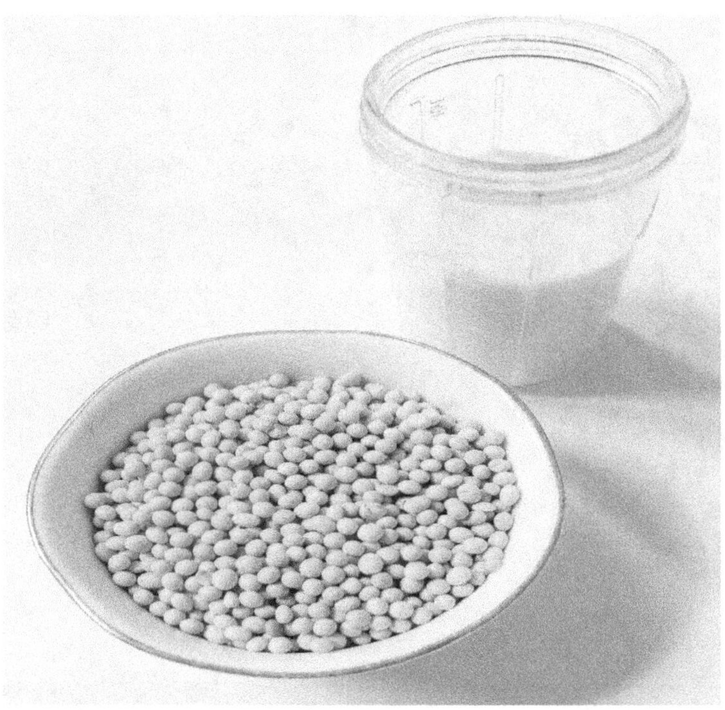

Tofu

You may incorporate soy in your diet in a variety of ways. One of them is tofu, a great alternative that packs nine grams of protein into a 3-ounce portion. Tofu is a heart-healthy food since it contains little saturated fat and cholesterol. It also contains essential nutrients including iron, calcium, and important amino acids. You can use tofu in a lot of different dishes, such as salads, soups, and stir-fries. Its mild flavor allows it to absorb flavors and spices, making it an excellent accent to any culinary recipe.

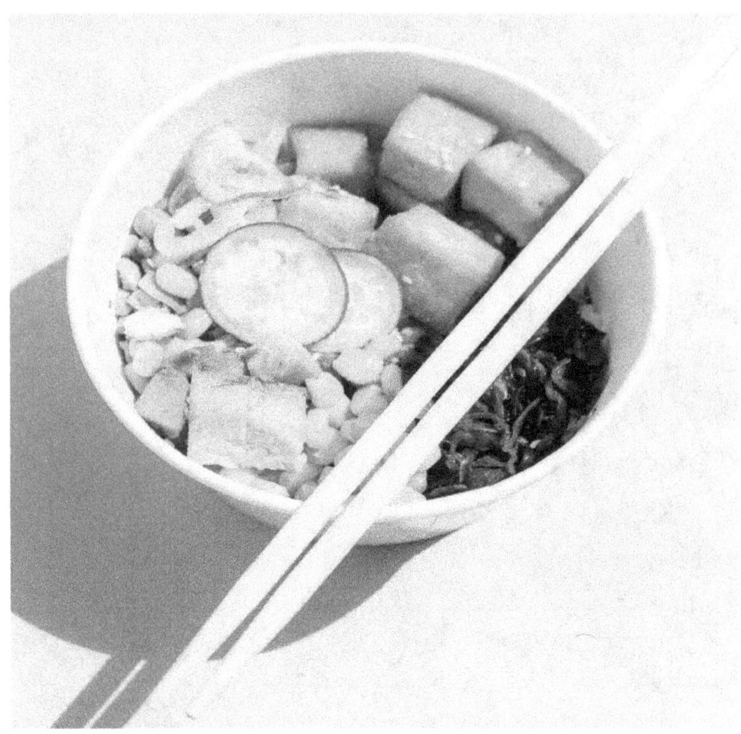

Quinoa

Quinoa is a multipurpose seed that is available in red, black, white, and blended colors. These seeds are not only tasty but also abundant in calories for vegetarians. For 100g meal, cooked quinoa provides more than 4g of protein. Since quinoa contains all 22 of the essential amino acids that our bodies require, it is thought to be the greatest plant-based protein source. In addition, quinoa is a wonderful source of minerals, vitamins, and dietary fiber.

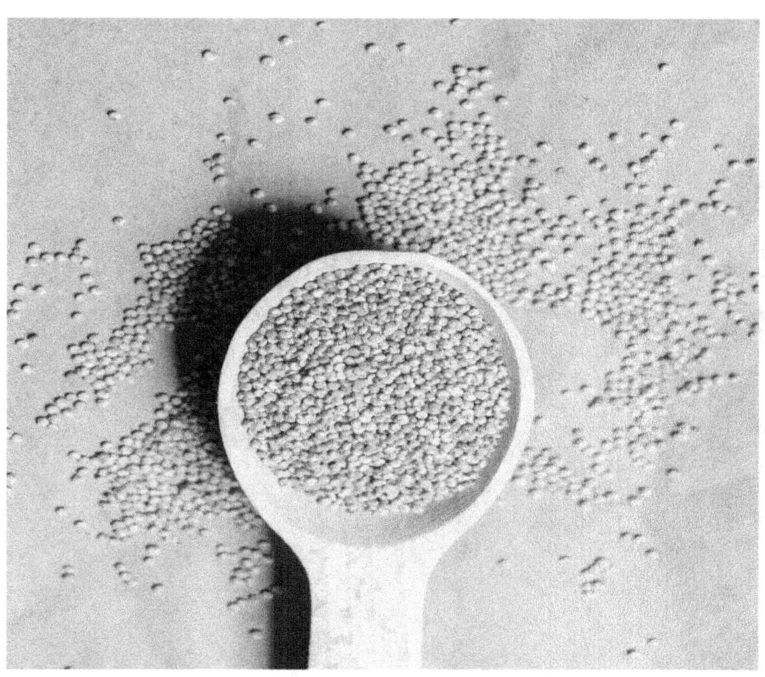

Chia seeds

Chia seeds have a high protein concentration despite their small size. A teaspoon of chia seeds provides about 2g of protein. These nutritious seeds can be added to various recipes to increase their protein value. Your food' nutritional content and texture can both be enhanced with chia seeds. You can therefore include them in your regular diet if you're looking for the greatest vegetarian protein diet.

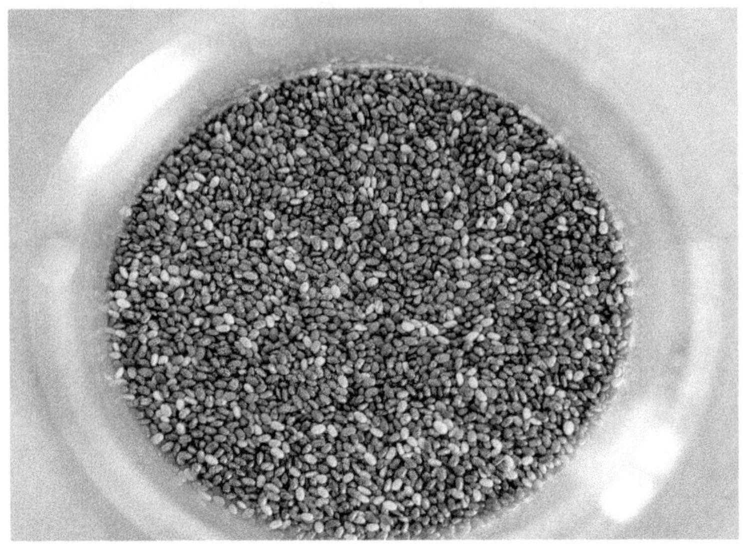

Flax Seeds

Flax seeds are little, delicious seeds with a host of health advantages. They offer a decent quantity of natural protein per meal, making them great options for vegetarians. Flax seeds are high in fiber, vitamins, minerals, and important omega-3 fatty acids in addition to protein. These nutrient-dense seeds can be consumed in a number of ways, including ground flaxseed or flaxseed oil.

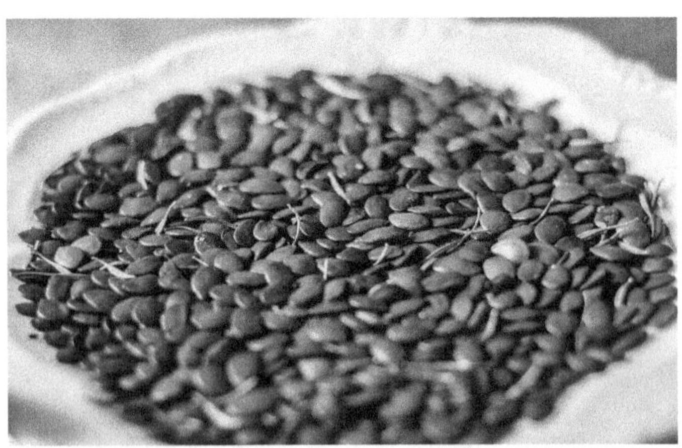

Sesame seeds

There are very nutrient-dense little seeds. They contain a lot of protein, which our bodies need to create and repair tissues. With a vegetarian or vegan diet, sesame seeds can help you get extra protein in your diet. To add crunch and nutrients to salads or baked goods, sprinkle sesame seeds on top.

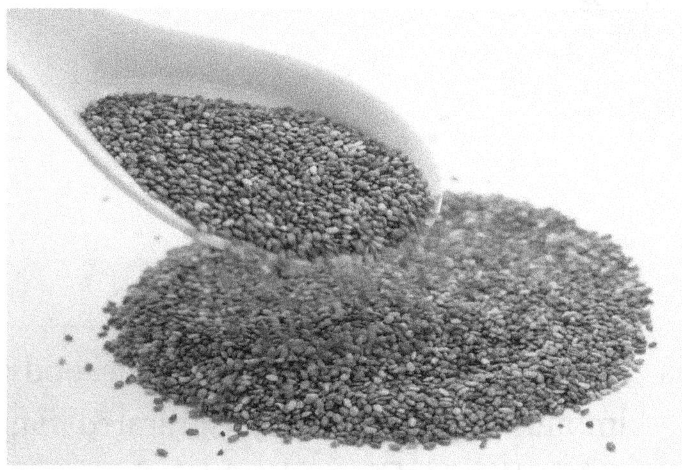

Sprouts

Eating sprouts can provide you with several health benefits and is a great way to get plant-based protein. Because small, young plants are so full of essential nutrients and enzymes, they are extraordinarily healthy. Amino acids, which are essential for muscle growth, healing, and general bodily function, are also abundant in sprouts. They are simple to digest and provide a full protein profile. You may meet your daily protein needs by incorporating these little protein powerhouses into your meals.

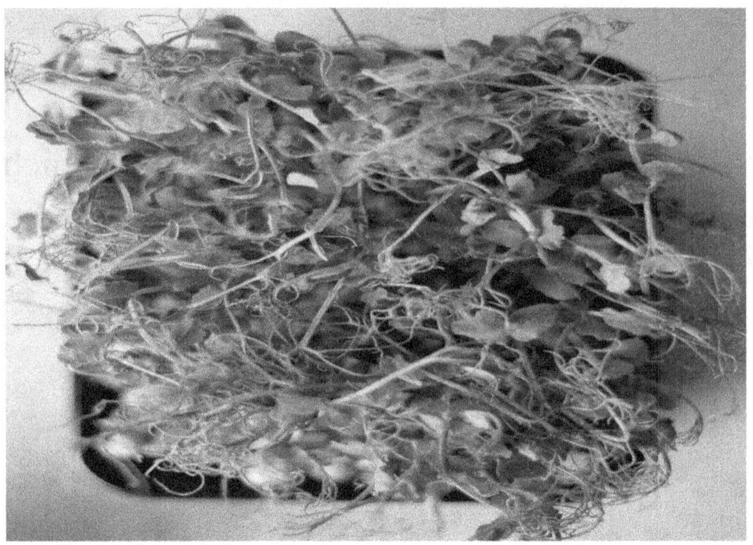

Almonds

The finest vegetarian fat source is almonds, which also give your body critical nutrients including protein. Almonds include monounsaturated fats that are good for the heart. You can get the benefits of healthy fats from almonds and still meet your protein needs. As a result, to include protein in a vegetarian diet, you should include almonds in your breakfast routine.

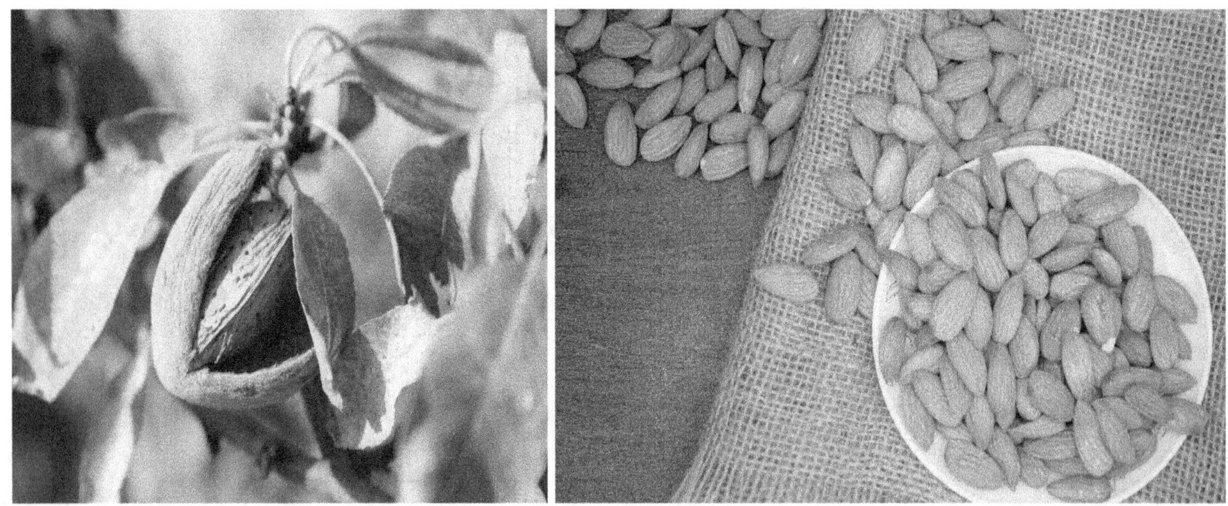

Pistachios

Another high-protein, health-promoting option for vegetarians are pistachios. They have the same monounsaturated fats, fiber, vitamins, and minerals as almonds. Pistachios can enhance sensations of fullness, support healthy cholesterol levels, and enhance digestion. However, because they are high in calories, it's crucial to pay attention to portion proportions.

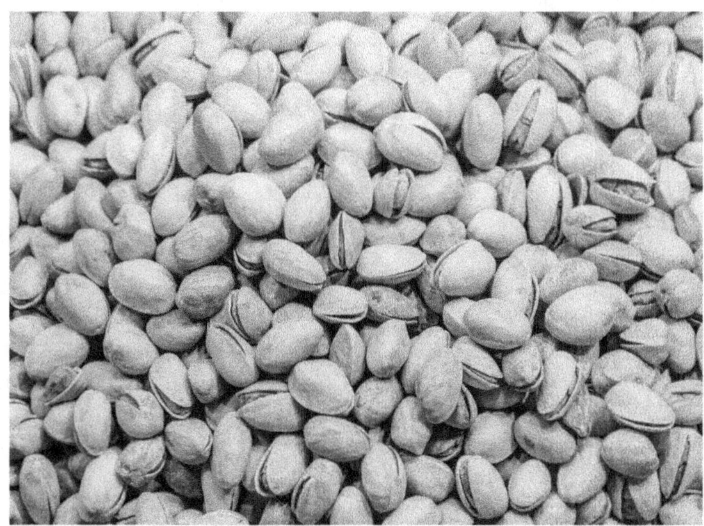

Broccoli

Broccoli is a fantastic choice for anyone searching for plant-based protein substitutes because it provides a decent amount of protein despite being a vegetable. Broccoli has little calories and a high nutritional content, including fiber, vitamins, and minerals. Broccoli helps ease constipation and aid with digestion. Additionally, it has a wealth of vitamins and minerals that support a robust immune system. Broccoli also protects against cancer and heart disease. So, if you want to eat a tasty and healthful dinner, broccoli should be on your diet.

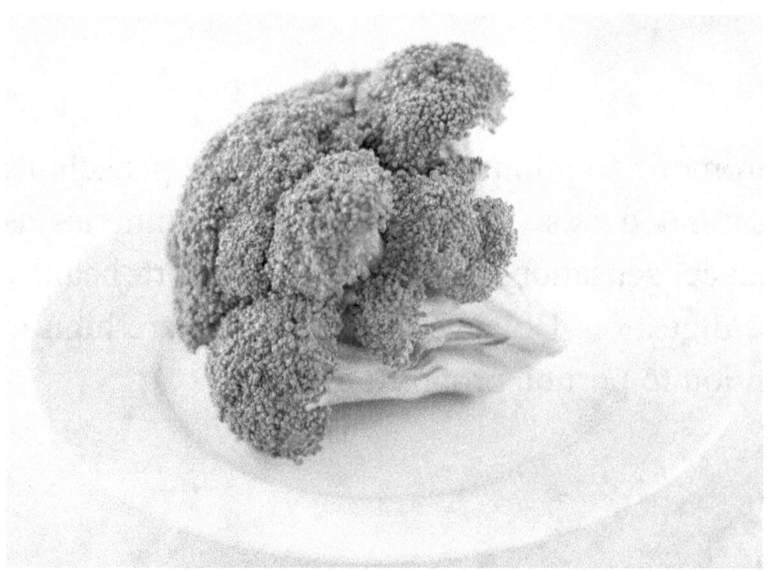

Spinach

This leafy green vegetable has an abundance of vital vitamins and minerals in addition to providing a substantial amount of protein. In addition, spinach is strong in fiber and low in calories, which promotes fullness and aids with digestion. Spinach also contains high amounts of calcium, iron, vitamin C, and other beneficial elements. Spinach is delicious as a side dish, in stir-fries, and in salads.

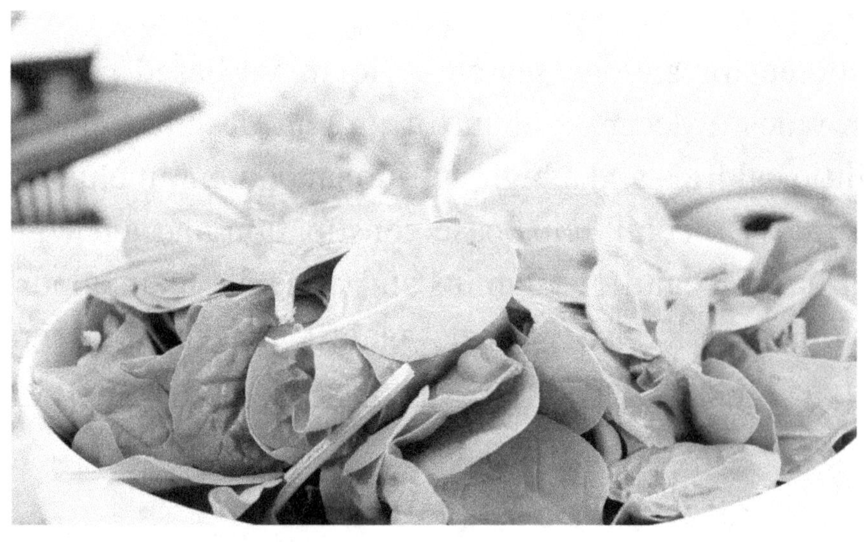

Pumpkin seeds

One of the best and healthiest sources of plant protein is pumpkin seeds. In addition to healthy fats, fiber, vitamins, and minerals, it has a high protein content. These include omega-3 fatty acids, iron, zinc, and magnesium, all of which promote different body processes. Antioxidant properties are another well-known benefit of pumpkin seeds. It can shield your cells from the harm that free radicals can do.

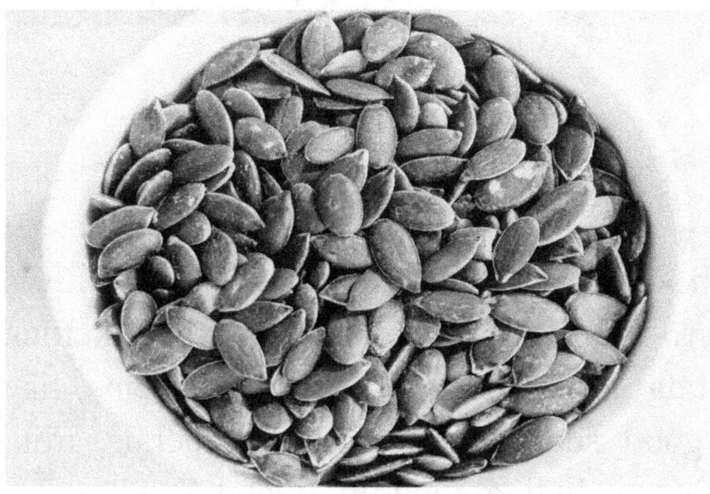

Ragi

Finger millet, often known as ragi, is considered to be one of the greatest plant-based protein sources. Compared to other grains, ragi provides higher protein per serving, making it a wonderful supplement to a vegan diet. It also contains high levels of vitamins, minerals, and fiber, such as calcium, iron, and magnesium. It can be eaten in a variety of forms, including baked goods, pancakes, and porridge.

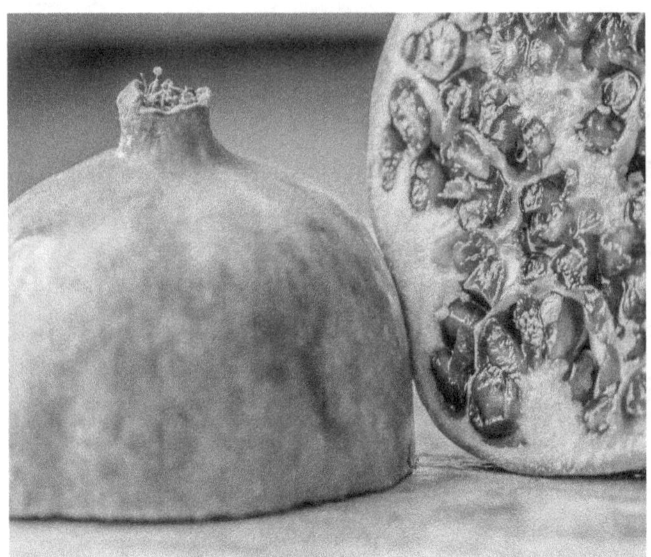
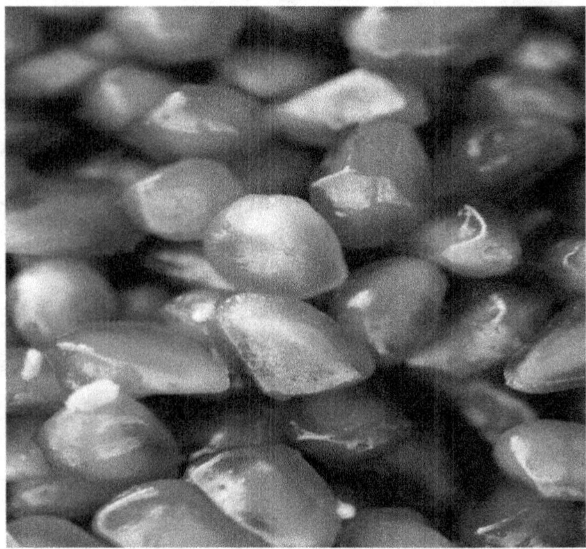

Wheat germ

One of the best sources of protein for a plant-based diet is wheat germ. It is the densely nutrient-packed embryo found in the center of a wheat kernel. Wheat germ is tiny, but it's bursting at the seams with vital nutrients, like protein. Wheat germ is also a good source of vitamins, minerals, iron, magnesium, fiber, and healthy fats including vitamin E and B vitamins.

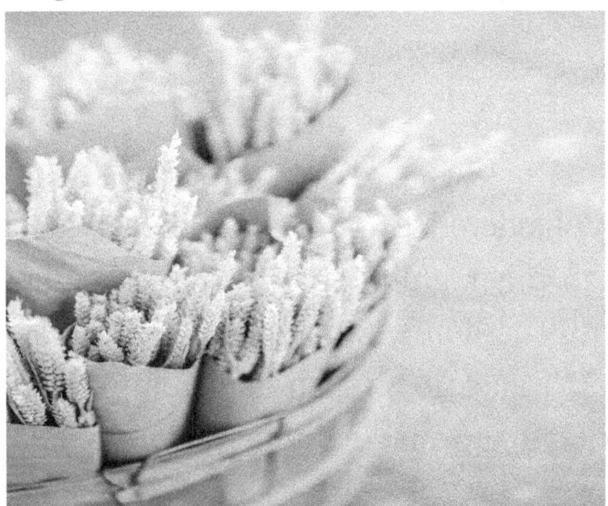
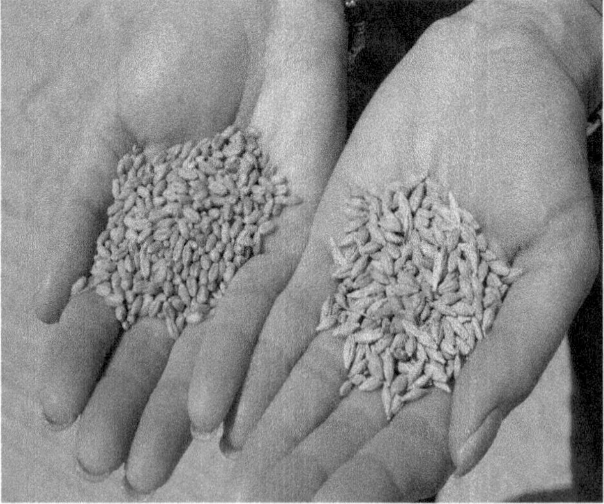

Buckwheat

Buckwheat is actually a seed, despite being called wheat. Its substantial protein content makes it advantageous for vegetarians seeking high-protein vegetarian meals. The antioxidants in buckwheat help lower the risk of heart disease and diabetes. In addition to being gluten-free, buckwheat is a fantastic option for anyone with celiac disease or gluten sensitivity.

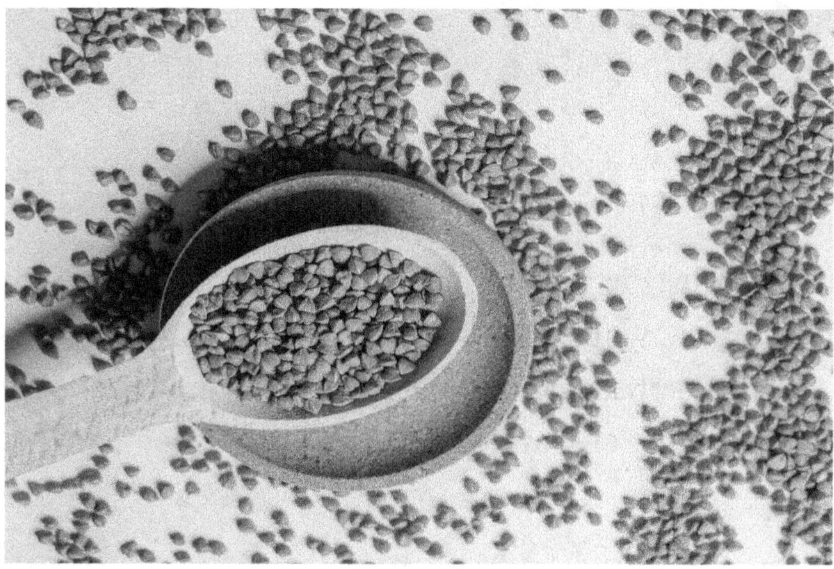

Jowar

You should eat jowar if you're searching for a gluten-free protein source. For vegans, these grains are a good source of protein. It has vital amino acids that your body needs to repair damaged tissues. Jowar can aid with digestion, provide you sustained energy, and enhance your general health. You can rap the health benefits of jowar by eating its porridge or rotis.

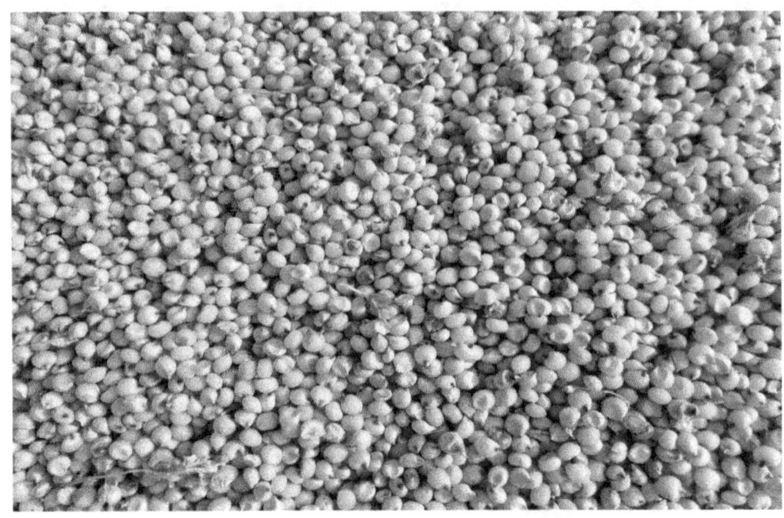

Mushrooms

The greatest foods high in protein for vegetarians are mushrooms, so you may include them in your diet as well. Due to their low calorie and fat content, mushrooms are a healthy substitute for weight loss. They are also a fantastic source of minerals, vitamins, and antioxidants, all of which support health.

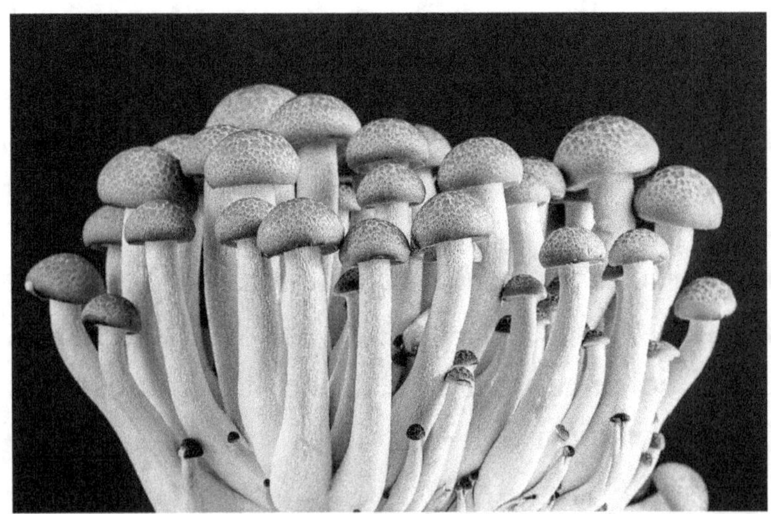

There are many options available, regardless of whether you lead a vegan lifestyle or just want to increase the amount of plant-based protein in your diet. You can leave a better lifestyle by including plant-based protein sources in your diet. So unleash your inner chef and discover the amazing world of plant-based protein!

Crucial Amino Acids for the Repair of Muscle

Muscle healing is a vital encore in the complex dance of sports performance. The building blocks of protein, essential amino acids, are crucial to this process because they help your muscles get stronger, regenerate, and mend after every activity. Come along with us as we delve into the world of vital amino acids and uncover the keys to faster muscle repair in the context of vegan sports.

Amino Acids' Function in Muscle Repair

Explore the underlying essential amino acids and how important they are for muscle repair. Learn how these small molecules support overall muscle health, discomfort in the muscles, and aid in the synthesis of proteins. Discover the special advantages that every necessary amino acid—from leucine to lysine—brings to the recuperation phase.

Sources of Essential Amino Acids from Plants

Learn about the abundance of plant-based sources that supply every important amino acids your body needs. Explore the range of plant-powered choices that guarantee you get the full spectrum of amino acids to support the best possible muscle repair, from quinoa and tofu to hemp seeds and beyond.

The Benefit of Leucine

Focus on leucine, one of the most important and potent amino acids. Discover how leucine is essential for athletes looking to improve muscle growth and recovery since it plays a critical function in promoting muscle protein synthesis. Examine plant sources high in leucine and recipes that maximizes its benefits.

Branched-chain amino acids BCAAs

Discover the advantages of valine, isoleucine, and leucine—branched-chain amino acids. Examine the ways in which BCAAs aid in muscle repair, lessen the damage that exercise causes to muscles, and lesen weariness after extended activity. Accept the power of these necessary amino acids by consuming them in natural food sources or as supplements made from plants.

When to Take Amino Acids for Recuperation

When it comes to consuming amino acids to aid in muscle regeneration, timing is crucial. To get the most out of vital amino acids, find out when is the best time to eat them. Find out how to effectively include amino acids into your vegan athlete lifestyle, from pre-workout methods to post-workout rituals.

Increase Your Amino Acid Intake

Master the kitchen with meals that will increase your intake of critical amino acids. Discover delectable ways to boost muscle regeneration while delighting your taste buds, from smoothies rich in amino acids to savory recipes that blend complementing plant proteins.

Supplements that Support Amino Acids

Explore the world of plant-powered amino acid supplements and find choices that fit your lifestyle. Examine how these additions, which range from plant-based protein powders to particular amino acid supplements, can offer focused assistance for improved muscle repair.

Amino Acids and the Prevention of Injury

Examine how important amino acids contribute to the prevention and treatment of injuries. Recognize how keeping your amino acid levels at appropriate levels can help your muscles, tendons, and connective tissues remain resilient, lowering your chance of injury and promoting long-term athletic success.

Adapting Your Amino Acid Consumption to Your Objectives

Adjust the amount of amino acids you consume to your specific sports objectives. Whether your goals are endurance, strength training, or a mix of the two, learn how to customize your amino acid regimen to improve your results and develop more quickly.

Explore the complex world of vital amino acids in this chapter, and see how incorporating them wisely into your vegan athlete lifestyle can be the secret to unmatched muscle building and recovery. It's time to master the science of amino acids and reach new heights in your athletic career.

High-Voltage Sources of Carbohydrates

The unsung heroes of athletic energy, carbohydrates give you the energy you need to power through each workout, practice, and competition. Using high-energy carbohydrate sources becomes essential for vegan athletes to maintain endurance and reach their maximum potential. Discover the boundless energy that comes from plant-powered carbs by traveling with us into their bright universe.

The Energy Dance: The Role of Carbs in Sports Performance

Examine how carbs function as an athlete's main source of energy. Recognize how these macronutrients are transformed into glucose, which powers your body and mind as you exercise. Every stage of your athletic journey requires carbohydrates, from quick spurts of intensity to sustainment.

Whole Grains: The Basis for Energy Produced by Plants

Discover the abundant realm of whole grains, where fiber, vitamins, and minerals are abundantly found in carbohydrates that are high in energy. Discover how these healthful grains—from oats and barley to brown rice and quinoa—offer a consistent energy release that will bolster your workouts and enhance your general well-being.

Root vegetables and sweet potatoes: sources of natural energy

Discover the energy reserve buried beneath the ground. Carrots, beets, and sweet potatoes are full of flavor and nutrients, but they are also high in complex carbs, which provide a continuous energy source. Discover how to incorporate these root veggies into your pre-workout fueling regimen.

Fruits that Boost Energy

Take a fruit-filled trip and explore a variety of fruits that can be used as high-energy sources of carbohydrates. Discover how the natural sugars found in fruits and vegetables—from bananas and berries to mangoes and oranges—provide rapid energy increases that make them ideal for pre-workout snacks and on-the-go nutrition.

Legumes: Protein-Pumping Carbohydrate Powerhouses

Review legumes in light of carbohydrates. Legumes are well known for their high protein content, but they also provide a significant amount of complex carbs. Explore recipes that highlight the double advantages of legumes: they provide energy and nutrients that help develop muscle.

Bread, Pasta, and More: Savoring Carbs for a Reason

Savor the delights of bread, pasta, and other grains. Discover how to select whole grain products that can improve your athletic performance in addition to satisfying your demand for carbohydrates. Find recipes that transform basic staples into meals that are packed with energy for athletes.

Energy Bars and Dried Fruits: Convenient Source of Carbohydrate Energy

Discover the portability of energy bars and dried fruits as sources of high-energy carbs. Check out how these snacks may become your go-to companions for sustaining energy while you're on the go, whether you're refueling on a long run or need a fast pick-me-up in between workouts.

Strategies for Endurance Athletes Using Carb Loading

Examine the idea of carb loading for long-duration sports. Learn the concepts behind deliberately upping your carbohydrate intake prior to a competition in order to optimize your glycogen stores and guarantee that you have the energy reserve required for a prolonged physical effort.

Maintaining a Carbohydrate Balance for Best Results

Recognize the subtleties of carbohydrates balancing for peak sports performance. Be it long-distance running or high-intensity interval training, discover how to adjust your carbohydrate intake to suit the needs of your training program and the sport you've chosen.

You will explore the world of high-energy carb sources and uncover a variety of tastes and textures that will enhance your vegan lifestyle while providing fuel for your workouts. It's time to reject the energy that carbohydrates derived from plants provide for your sports pursuits.

Chapter 3: Power-Packed Breakfasts

Energizing Smoothie Bowls

Discover the colorful and nourishing world of reviving smoothie bowls to elevate your morning routines and pre-workout regimens. These bowls, full with a symphony of tastes, nutrients, and plant-powered energy, are a celebration of the goodness that powers your day, not simply a meal. Come learn the artistry of creating vibrant smoothie bowls that will tantalize your taste buds and give your vegan athlete lifestyle a serious boost.

Smoothie Bowls' Beauty

Discover the appeal of smoothie bowls as a creative and nutritious blank canvas. Learn how adding fruits, veggies, and plant-based proteins can turn an ordinary breakfast into a visually spectacular, high-injector.

Basic Components: Establishing the Base

Discover the fundamental components that form the basis of the ideal smoothie bowl. Learn how these ingredients produce a creamy and pleasant texture while providing a quick energy boost, from frozen fruits and veggies to plant-based yogurt and nut butters.

Additions Packed with Protein

Upgrade your smoothie bowl with high-protein ingredients that help you reach your fitness objectives. Discover how to add the nutrients your bowl needs for long-lasting energy and muscle recovery, from hemp hearts to chia seeds and plant-based protein powders.

Superfood Boosts: Every Spoonful Contains Nutrients

Explore the realm of superfood boosters to transform your smoothie bowl into an incredibly nutrient-dense meal. Discover how these superfoods, which range from goji berries and acai to maca powder and spirulina, can improve both your general health and sports performance.

Liquid Remedies: The Ideal Combination

Learn how to make the ideal liquid elixir to mix in your smoothie bowl. Discover how various liquids, such as almond milk, coconut water, green tea, and fruit juices, can improve the nutritional content and flavor of your bowl.

Creative Garnishes: Explosion of Flavor and Texture

Use visually striking toppings that add taste and texture to transform your smoothie bowl into a work of art. Learn to build a visually appealing and gratifying bowl that satisfies all your senses, filled with everything from crunchy granola and nuts to fresh fruits and edible flowers.

Seasonal Inspirations: Appreciating the Abundance of Nature

Enjoy the abundance of nature as you embrace the changing seasons with these smoothie bowl inspirations. To connect with the freshness and vitality of the ingredients around you, try recipes that showcase seasonal fruits and flavors.

Personalizing Your Bowl: Adapting to Your Preferences

Gain the skills to personalize your smoothie bowl to your preferences and dietary requirements. Learn how to modify your bowl to meet your unique goals, whether you're aiming for a post-workout recuperation or an energy boost prior to your session.

Smoothie Bowl Recipes: Suitable for Any Event

Take a tour through a variety of revitalizing smoothie bowl recipes that are appropriate for every occasion. Learn about a variety of delectable recipes that suit your vegan athlete lifestyle, from breakfast bowls to post-workout bowls that revitalize you.

Photographic Advice for Smoothie Bowls

Discover how to use photography to convey the visual attractiveness of your smoothie bowls. Discover easy ways to highlight the beauty of your creations, transforming your smoothie bowls into eye-catching visual treats for Instagram or personalized mementos.

By exploring the world of nutritious smoothie bowls, you'll not only fuel your body but also develop delight and creativity in your cooking. It's time to upgrade your vigan athletic lifestyle, one spoonful at a time, by embracing the art of blending and bowl building.

Protein-Rich Waffles and Pancakes

Pancakes and waffles are cozy, protein-packed delights that can transform your breakfast rituals. These plant-powered innovations give your body the necessary protein it needs while also pleasing your taste. Take a culinary adventure with us as we delve into the art of making protein-rich pancakes and waffles that will give your vegan lifestyle a twist.

Waffles and Pancakes: An Allure

Learn why waffles and pancakes are breakfast staples that never go out of style. Recognize the happiness these fluffy treats offer to your morning routine and how they are used as flexible canvases to incorporate plant-based protein sources throughout your day.

Flour Power: Selecting an Appropriate Base

Discover the range of flours that go into making your high-protein pancakes and waffles. Explore the distinct aromas and textures that each type of flour—from almond and chickpea flour to whole wheat and oat flour—brings to your morning meal.

Proteins from Plants: Boosting Your Batter

Add plant-based proteins to your batter to aid with muscle repair and long-term energy. Discover how adding protein-rich nuts and seed butters, silken tofu, and plant-based yogurt can improve the nutritional profile of your pancakes and waffles.

Liquid Harmony: Integral Components Combined

Explore the world of liquid ingredients to make the ideal balance for your waffle and pancake batter. Learn how these liquids—which range from fruit purées and aquafaba to almond and coconut milk—contribute to a smooth, pourable consistency.

Flavors and Sweeteners: Harmonizing the Taste

Achieve the ideal harmony between taste and sweetness in your high-protein dishes. Examine natural sweeteners like agave nectar and maple syrup, and learn how to enhance the flavor and depth of your pancakes and waffles with spices and extracts.

Egg Substitutes: Veganizing the Traditional Recipes

Learn about vegan substitutes for regular eggs that bind and leaven pancakes and waffles. Discover how to achieve the ideal texture without sacrificing flavor with these egg substitutes, which range from commercial egg replacers to flax and chia eggs.

Ingenious Add-Ons: Texture and Enhanced Nutrient Content

Use inventive add-ins to give your pancakes and waffles more texture and nutrients. Discover how these additives, which range from chopped nuts and seeds to dried fruits and grated veggies, provide layers of flavor and nutritious richness.

Cooking Methods: Reaching the Optimal Texture

To get the ideal texture, become an expert pancake and waffle cook. Discover how to get golden exteriors and fluffy innards so that every bite is a pleasurable experience.

Protein-Rich Toppings: The Final Element

Top your protein-rich concoctions with a variety of delectable toppings to complete them. Discover how to add the last touches that transform your pancakes and waffles into a visual and gastronomic treat, from fresh fruit and nut butters to plant-based whipped cream and syrups.

Recipes to Satisfy Every Want

Take a culinary trip with these assortment of high-protein pancake and waffle recipes that will fulfill all of your cravings. Discover a variety of breakfast options that suit your vegan athlete lifestyle, from traditional stacks to creative taste combinations.

As you dive into the realm of high-protein pancakes and waffles, you'll improve breakfast and give your mornings the fuel they need for long-lasting energy and peak performance in the gym. Now is the time to turn, pile, and enjoy the goodness of plant-based breakfasts.

Variations of Overnight Oats

Overnight oats are so simple and versatile that epeн will revolutionize your morning routine. These delicious dishes are a great way to showcase a variety of flavors, textures, and nutrient-dense foods, in addition to providing a quick and easy breakfast option. Come along on a journey through the process of creating varieties of overnight oats that suit your taste buds and support your vegan athletic lifestyle.

Why Overnight Oats Are Appealing

Learn why overnight oats are becoming a popular breakfast option. Discover the enchantment that ensures when basic components, after soaking overnight, become a creamy and delectable morning treat. Discover the health advantages and east of use that have made overnight oats a go-to meal for vegan athletes.

Oat Base: Selecting the Appropriate Base

Discover the range of oats that you can use as the base for your variants on overnight oats. Learn how different varieties of oats affect the texture and consistency of your breakfast bowl, from traditional rolled oats to steel-cut oats and gluten-free choices.

Fluid Components: Producing Smooth Harmony

Explore the world of liquid ingredients that give your overnight oats a creamy, delicious flavor. Learn how these beverages, which range from plant-based yogurt and almond or coconut milk to fruit juices and almond milk, add to a delicious and fulfilling meal.

Flavor enhancers and sweeteners: Customizing Taste Use a range of sweeteners and flavor enhancers to balance sweetness and add layers of flavor to your overnight oats. To make a bowl that pleases the palate, experiment with spices, extracts, and superfoods in addition to exploring natural sweeteners like agave nectar and maple syrup.

Protein-Rich Supplements: Energy-Dense

Add some plant-based ingredients to your overnight oats to boost their protein level. Discover how these additions, which range from nut butters and seeds to fruits high in protein and plant-based protein powders, support continuous energy and muscle recovery.

Texture and Crispness: Ingenious Add-Ons

Add some inventive mix-ins to your overnight oats to give them crunch and an extra nutritional boost. Find out how adding chopped nuts and granola, or dried fruits and cocoa nibs, improves the breakfast bowl's sensory appeal.

Sweet Treats: Overflowing with Vibrant Juiciness

Discover the variety of delicious fruits that can enhance the natural sweetness and freshness of your overnight oats. Learn how seasonal and exotic fruits may elevate your morning bowl from sliced bananas and berries to citrus and tropical fruits.

Superfoods Packed with Nutrients: Increasing Health Benefits

Add nutrient-dense superfoods to your overnight oats to increase their health benefits. See the variety of superfoods that support your health, from goji berries and hemp hearts to chia seeds and flaxseeds.

Creative Layering: Artistry in a Jar Embrace the creative layering in a jar as an artistic endeavor. Discover how to make visually beautiful overnight oats by layering various components to produce a breakfast masterpiece that will look amazing.

Dishes to Suit Every Taste: Take your taste buds on a culinary journey with our assortment of overnight oats recipes. Make your mornings exciting and nourishing with our repertoire of breakfast delights, which range from traditional combos to creative flavor fusions.

You'll streamline your morning routine and infuse your vegan lifestyle with some creativity and flavor as you dive into the world of overnight oats variations. Now is the perfect time to enjoy the countless benefits of overnight oats and begin your mornings with a bowl of healthy delight.

Chapter 4: Nourishing Lunches

Lentil and Quinoa Power Bowls

The powerful combination of quinoa and lentils in a symphony of flavors, textures, and nutrient-rich ingredients will up your lunch or supper game. These plant-powered bowls are a great way to fuel your vigan athletic lifestyle in addition to making a filling and substantial meal. Come along on a gastronomic journey as we delve into the technique of creating power bowls made with quinoa and lentils that will both satisfy your hunger and nourishe your body.

Lentils with Quinoa, the Power Couple

Learn how to use the power couple of lentils and quinoa as the base for your power bowls. Learn about the health advantages of these high-protein components and how their contrasting textures combine to produce a filling, well-balanced supper.

Quinoa Types: Going Beyond the Fundamentals

Investigate the many quinoa types to bring some variety to your power bowls. Learn how each kind of quinoa, from black and white to red and white to tri-color blends, adds a distinct texture and eye-catching appearance to your culinary creations.

A Spectrum of Colors in Lentil Varieties

Explore the universe of lentil types that help your power bowel color scheme. Discover how different lentil kinds, such as, black, and brown, give unique flavors and textures to enhance the vibrancy and flavor of your bowls.

Cooking Methods: Optimal Quinoa and Lentil Cooking

Learn how to cook lentils and quinoa to absolute perfection. Discover various cooking techniques and pick up some insider knowledge to get the perfect texture for your power bowls, guaranteeing that each bite is satisfying and full of nutrition.

Tasty Soups with Spices: Enhancing Flavor

To improve the flavor of your power bowls, add savory broths and seasonings to your quinoa and lentils. Learn how these additions, which range from savory vegetable broths to aromatic herbs and spices, give your plant-based recipes more depth and complexity.

Proteins Driven by Plants: Increasing Density of Nutrients

Plant-powered proteins will help your power bowls have a higher nutritious density. Discover how these protein options, which range from chickpeas and edamame to tempeh and tofu, can improve the satisfaction and ability of your quinoa and lentil bowls to nourish your muscles.

Vibrant Vegetables: A Visual Treat

Use vibrant, high-nutrient vegetables to make your power bowls and eye-catching visual feast. Learn to balance textures and flavors in your bowls with everything from roasted sweet potatoes and cherry tomatoes to leafy greens and bell peppers.

Final Flourish: Nutrient-Rich Toppings

Add a final flourish to your quinoa and lentil power bowls by adding nutrient-rich toppings. Discover how various toppings, such as avocado slices, crunchy nuts, tahini drizzles, and balsamic glazes, improve the overall flavor and presentation of your dishes.

Balanced Macros: Preparing Bowls Packed with Nutrients

Recognize the fundamentals of balanced macronutrients when creating power bowls that are high in nutrients. Discover how to thoughtfully mix meats, veggies, lentils, quinoa, and toppings to make a filling meal that complements your vegan athletic lifestyle.

Appetizers for All Tastes

Take a culinary adventure with our assortment of power bowl recipes including quinoa and lentils that are sure to please any kind of palate. Discover a variety of filling and tasty dishes that make plant-powered eating an interesting experience, from bowls with Mediterranean influences to dishes with Asian influences.

As you dive into the world of power bowls made with quinoa and lentils, you'll not only enjoy tasty meals but also provide your body with a wide range of nutrients that are critical for optimal athletic performance. Now is the time to make bowls that invigorate and nourish, giving a plant-powered burst of vitality to your table.

Vegan Sandwiches and Wraps

Experience the rich and varied world of vegan sandwiches and wraps as you go on a voyage of portable pleasures. These plant-powered recipes, which range from light and refreshing wraps to filling and substantial sandwiches, provide a tasty and easy approach to support your vegan athlete lifestyle. Come learn how to make sandwiches and wraps that will improve the flavor and nutritional value of your on-the-go meals.

The Convenient Treat: Sandwiches and Wraps

Experience the delight of on-the-go meals with our vegan sandwiches and wraps. Discover how these recipes' adaptability and ease make them ideal for picnics, last-minute lunches, and post-workout feeding.

Tie It Up: Selecting the Ideal Tie

Take a look at the assortment of wrappers that may hold your vegan treats. Know how different wraps can improve the texture and overall feel of your wraps and sandwiches, from classic tortillas to gluten-free options like rice paper and collard greens.

Tasty Spreads & Hummus: The Foundation

Using hummus and tasty spreads, create a delectable base layer for your wraps and sandwiches. Find out how these spreads give your portable dishes depth and richness, from the traditional hummus and avocado spread to the vegan cream cheese.

Plant-Powered Proteins: The Complementary Base

Provide a strong base of plant-based proteins for your sandwiches and wraps. Discover the range of protein options that give your portable dishes body and satisfaction, from marinated tofu and tempeh to chickpea salad and seitan.

Crisp & Vibrant Fresh Vegetables and Greens

Mix in some fresh veggies and greens to give your wraps and sandwiches some crunch and color. Discover how these components, which range from crunchy bell peppers and shredded carrots to crisp lettuce and juicy tomatoes, add to a pleasant and well-balanced taste.

Ingenious Fillings: Going Above and Beyond

Transform your sandwiches and wraps with inventive fillings that go beyond the norm. Discovery novel taste combinations that give every bit a satisfying crunch, from roasted sweet potatoes and apple slices to pickled veggies and sauteed mushrooms.

Strong Tastes: Spices, Herbs, and Sauces

Use sauces, herbs, and spices to add robust flavors to your sandwiches and wraps. Learn how these ingredients, which range from fiery sriracha and tahini to aromatic basil and cilantro, improve the flavor profile of your portable dishes.

Baking, Grilling, or Raw: Methods of Cooking

Try experimenting with different cooking methods to improve the flavor and texture of your sandwiches and wraps. Discover how to use each cooking technique to make a variety of tasty and portable meals, regardless of whether you prefer raw, baked, or grilled ingredients.

Carry-Along Sandwiches and Wraps: Quick and Easy Choices

Make your sandwiches and wraps portable by customizing them. Learn tricks and recipes that will keep your handheld creations mess-free and portable—perfect for travel, hectic days, or outdoor activities.

Recipes to Satisfy Every Want

With a variety of vegan wrap and sandwich recipes to satisfy any craving, you may have a gastronomic journey. Find a variety of portable traits that make plant-powered eating enticing and tasty, from robust stacked sandwiches to wraps with a Mediterranean influence.

You will discover a world of tasty, portable plant-powered meals and reinvent the concept of plant-powered, on-the-go dining as you explore the world of vegan wraps and sandwiches. It's time to put a bow on it and savor the goodness with portable products that support your busy lifestyle.

Plant-Based Proteins Boost Salads' Vitality

Plant-based protein will turn your salad experience into a colorful, energy-danse fast. These nutrient-dense salads provide you the necessary fuel for your vigan athletic lifestyle in addition to serving as a cool and filling lunch. Learn how to create vibrant salads that highlight the benefits of plant-based proteins.

The Plant-Powered Protein Edition of The Salad Revival

Take a stab at reviving salads by adding plant-based proteins. Learn how these high-protein components transform salads from light side dishes to filling and stimulating main courses that make for a delightful and fulfilling meal.

High-Protein Greens: The Basis of Salads

Start your salad with greens high in protein that are high in nutrients and freshness. Discover how leafy greens, which range from kale and spinach to arugula and watercress, make a colorful and nutrient-rich foundation for your invigorating salads.

Plant Protein Powerhouses: Legumes Abundant

Explore the world of legumes, the powerhouses of plant protein. Discover how these adaptable ingredients—from lentils and edamame to chickpeas and black beans—add texture, flavor, and a significant protein boost to your energetic salads.

Delights of Tempeh and Tofu: Soy-Based Proteins

Add the deliciousness of tempeh and tofu, two soy-based proteins with distinct taste profiles and textures, to your salads. Learn how these components, which range from seasoned tempeh strips to grilled tofu cubes, become the stars of your plant-powered salad recipes.

Quinoa and Grains: Rich Additions of Nutrients

Add quinoa and other grains to your salads to increase their nutritional value. Discover the variety of grains like bulgur, quinoa, and farro that not only add plant-based proteins to your energetic salads, but also add a hearty and satisfying element.

Nuts and Seeds: Crispy Sources of Protein

Nuts and seeds up the protein level and give your salads a pleasant crunch. You can add nuts and seeds to your salads to improve their texture and nutritional content. Some examples of these nuts and seeds are walnuts, sunflower seeds, and almonds.

Flavored Infusions of Marinated Proteins

Add marinated proteins to your salads to enhance the flavor of each bite. Discover how to make simple salads into savory, filling meals using marinated tofu skewers, tempeh strips, and seasoned beans.

Natural Sweetness and Nutrients in Fresh Fruits

Fresh fruit's inherent sweetness and nutrition counterbalance the savory components of your salads. Discover how these ingredients, which range from sliced apples and mango cubes to juicy berries and citrus segments, improve the flavor profile and appearance of your vibrant salads.

Brightly Colored Vegetables: A Rainbow of Benefit

Incorporate a range of vibrant veggies into your invigorating salads to commemorate the rainbow of goodness. Learn how to include a variety of veggies for both visual and nutritional impact, from colorful bell peppers and cherry tomatoes to crunchy cucumbers and roasted root vegetables.

Garnishes and Dressings: Tasty Conclusions

Serve your vibrant salads with tasty vinaigrettes and dressings. Discover how these finishing touches, such as balsamic Dijon vinaigrette or zesty lemon tahini, bring your salads' disparate components together and enhance their overall flavor.

Balanced Macros: Creating Salads Packed with Nutrients

Learn how to make salads that are high in nutrients and contain a balance of macronutrients. Discover how to blend veggies, healthy fats, and protein-rich components to make salads that are not only pleasant to eat but also sustain your energy levels for an active lifestyle.

Recipes to Suit Any Taste

Take a culinary adventure with these assortment of vibrant salad dishes that are sure to please any palate. Discover a variety of salads that make eating plant-based a colorful and satisfying experience, from Asian-inspired quinoa salads to Mediterranean protein-packed bowls.

You'll rediscover the art of colorful, nutrient-dense dining as you delve into the realm of invigorating salads with plant-based proteins. You'll also enjoy tasty and fulfilling meals. Now is the time toss, combine, and savor the deliciousness of salads that support your vegan athletic way of living.

59

Chapter 5: Satisfying Dinners

Vegan Pasta Recipes with Protein

Savor the cozy comfort of spaghetti with a plant-based twist. We'll look at how to make plant-based protein pasta recipes in this chapter that will not only satiate your appetites but also provide a good source of plant-based nutrients. These recipes, which range from traditional favorites to creative inventions, highlight the richness and diversity that vegan proteins offer to the pasta-eating experience.

Pasta Delights: Vegetarian Version

Take a gastronomic adventure with our plant-based protein pasta meals, which will redefine the delights of this popular comfort food. Learn about the wide variety of plant-based proteins that may make your pasta dishes into filling, healthy dinners.

Pasta Varieties Packed with Protein

Look into high-protein pasta options to use as the best for your vegan recipes. Find out how these substitutes, which range from edamame and quinoa blends to pasta made with lentils and chickpeas, not only boost the protein level of your meals but also give them distinctive flavors and textures.

Bean-Based Sauces: Limelighting Legumes

Bean-based sauces that highlight the benefits of legumes might enhance your pasta-eating experience. Discover how these protein-rich sauces may elevate your vegan protein pasta recipes, from creamy white bean Alfredo to hearty red lentil Bolognese.

Tempeh and Tofu Revisions

Add the adaptability of tempeh and tofu to your pasta preparations. Find out how these soy-based proteins provide a delicious chewiness and absorb the flavors of your favorite sauces, from crumbled tempeh in a savory pesto to marinated tofu cubes in a spicy arrabbiata sauce.

Various Nut and Seed Pesto Recipes

Savor the abundance of nuts and seeds in a range of pesto recipes. Discover how these high-protein sauces, which range from the traditional basil and pine nut pesto to the daring kale and walnut pesto, enhance the complexity and nuttiness of your vegan protein pasta recipes.

Pasta Salads With Legumes

Add some beans to your pasta salads to make them protein powerhouses. Learn how these legume-infused pasta salads, which range from lentil penne to chickpea fusilli salads, become energizing and fulfilling meals that are ideal for picnics, lunches, or post-workout refueling.

Veggie-Based Sauces Packed with Protein

Discover the world of high-protein, plant-based sauces that will elevate your pasta recipes. Learn how these vegetable-focused sauces, such as spinach and artichoke marinara and roasted cauliflower Alfredo, give your pasta a filling and healthy base.

Blends of Quinoa and Grain: Hearty Textures

Quinoa and other grain blends give your pasta dishes substantial textures. Discover how adding grains to your vegan protein pasta dishes may improve their heartiness and nutritional value, using recipes like quinoa and mushroom stroganoff or farro and roasted vegetable primavera.

Marvels of Seitan and Jackfruit

Add the savory delights of jackfruit and seitan to your arsenal of pasta dishes. Explore how plant-based meat substitutes, such as seitan sausage and sun-dried tomato linguine, may enhance your recipes with a powerful flavor and meat texture. Try dishes like BBQ jackfruit mac 'n' cheese.

Flavor Fusions: International Inspirations

Take a gourmet trip with inventive fusions that draw inspiration from various global cuisines. Discover how different flavors blend together to celebrate a variety of global tastes with dishes like Mediterranean chickpea orzo and Thai-inspired peanut noodle bowls.

Balanced Macros: Preparing Foods High in Nutrients

Recognize the fundamentals of balanced macros while creating vegan protein pasta dishes that are high in nutrients. Discover how to put together a range of veggies, whole-grain pastas, and protein-rich sauces to make meals that will nourish your active lifestyle in addition to pleasing your palate.

Recipes to Satisfy Any Desire

With a variety of vegan protein pasta dishes to satisfy every craving, on a tasteful trip. Discover a repertoire of pasta dishes that make plant-based meals a pleasurable and protein-rich experience, ranging from hearty classics to bold and imaginative variations.

Discovering the world of plant-based protein pasta dishes will allow you to appreciate the diversity and depth that plant-based proteins offer to your pasta experience in addition to indulging in tasty and filling meals. Now is the perfect moment to swirl, savor, and relish the taste of vegan pasta dishes that support your vegan way of living.

Filling Bean and Grain Stews

Hearty grain and bean stew are a comfortable embrace that will warm your soul and nourish your body. This will cover the craft of making hearty, satisfying stews that are driven by plants and packed with healthful grains, beans, and a variety of veggies. These stews are a celebration of flavor and nutrition, whether they are cooked in aromatic bowls or boiling pots.

Stewpot Symphony: Elegance Driven by Plants

Take in the symphony of aromas that emerges from a stewpot full of substantial grains and beans. Experience the depth and richness that this elegant plant-based dish provides to your table, offering both nourishment and fulfillment.

Plenty of Grains: The Foundation for Hearty Stews

Discover the range of grains that make up your stews' substantial base. Learn how these healthful grains, which range from quinoa and brown rice to barley and farro, provide body, texture, and nutritional value to your plant-based dishes.

Bean Bonanza: Stars Packed with Protein

Give your stews a focal point of protein-rich legumes to calibrate a bean abundance. Explore the range of beans that not only provide your stews vital nutrients but also heartiness, such as kidney beans, black beans, chickpeas, and lentils.

Aromatics and Broths: Delectable Bases

Utilize a blend of aromatics and broths to create savory bases for your substantial stews of meat. Find out how these ingredients may produce a flavorful and delectable foundation for your stews, from sautéed onions and garlic to hearty vegetable broth and herb-infused mixtures.

Root Vegetables: Adding a Hearty Touch

Use a variety of root vegetables to infuse your stews with robust deliciousness. Discover how these earthy ingredients, which range from turnips and parsnips to carrots and sweet potatoes, provide both sweetness and depth to your plant-based recipes.

Leafy Greens: Supplements Packed with Nutrients

Add color and vibrancy to your stews by incorporating leafy greens that are high in nutrients. Learn how the vitamins and minerals that these greens—from kale and spinach to Swiss chard and collard greens—add to your steps to make them not only heart but also nutrient-dense.

Tangy Accents with Tomatoes and Simmered Sauces

Simmered sauces and tomatoes provide tangy touches to your stews. Discover how these ingredients may give your plant-powered stews depth and acidity, from crushed tomatoes and tomato paste to homemade tomato-based sauces.

Spices and Seasonings: The Alchemy of Cooking

Use a range of seasonings and spices to enhance the flavor profile of your heart stews and indulge in culinary alchemy. Find out how these ingredients, which range from warming spices like cumin and coriander to aromatic herbs like thyme and rosemary, create a symphony of flavors in your stews.

Hearty Grains and Variations on Bean Stew

Try a range of robust stews made with grains and beans that are tailored to suit a range of palates. Explore an assortment of recipes that turn every stew into a memorable and fulfilling meal, ranging from traditional lentil and quinoa stews to especially prepared black bean and veggie dishes.

One-Pot Marvels: Cooking Made Easy

Savor the east of cooking by preparing grains, beans, and veggies all in one pot with these one-pot marvels. Look into recipes that let the flavors blend and develop stronger while they simmer together, while also making cooking easier.

Magic of the Slow Cooker and Instant Pot

Use the power of Instant Pots and slow cookers to make tasty, hands-off grain and bean stews. Learn how kitchen tools simplify hearty cooking with everything from set-it-and-forget-it stews to quick and effective Instant Pot recipes.

Season-Perfect Recipes

Take a gastronomic adventure with robust grain and bean stew recipes, designed for every season. Discover a year-round repertory that keeps your plant-powered meal time fascinating and fulfilling, from light and refreshing summer varieties to hearty winter soups.

You'll delight in filling meals and the pleasure of fragrant bowls and boiling pots that add comfort and fulfillment to your table as you dive into the realm of substantial grain and bean stew. Now is the moment to ladle, taste, and revel in the heartiness of stews made with plant-based ingredients to support your vegan athletic lifestyle.

Stir-Fries as Easy and Packed with Nutrients

Learn the art of stir-frying and go on a culinary adventure of quick and delectable masterpieces. We'll delve into the realm of nutrient-dense stir-fries in this chapter, which not only provide a quick fix for hectic days but also deliver a powerful punch of plant-based goodness. These stir-fries, in their sizzling woks and colorful bowls, are a celebration of flavor and efficiency.

Stir-Fry Symphony: Tasteful Elegance in a Flash

Take in the symphony of frying pans and colorful veggies that epitomizes the skill of stir-frying. Explore the beauty of tasty, fast cooking—where richness of nutrient-dense ingredients is combined with efficiency.

Fast-Cooking Grains: The Rapid Foundation

Discover quick-cook grains that provide a quick and easy stir-fry basis. Learn how these grains, which range from bulgur and brown rice to quinoa and couscous, make a nutritious base for your nutrient-dense stir-fries.

Tempeh and Tofu Packed with Protein: Quick-Cooking Gems

Tofu and tempeh are fast-cooking heroes of stir-fries; up your game. Discover how plant-powered proteins, which range from crunchy tofu cubes to tempeh strips, swiftly absorb flavors and become the focal point of your nutrient-dense stir-fry masterpieces.

Colorful veggies: lively Crunch Use a rainbow of colorful veggies to give your stir-fries a lively crunch. Find out how these quick-cooking vegetables, which range from bell peppers and broccoli to snap peas and carrots, provide texture and visual appeal to your nutrient-dense stir-fries.

Leafy Greens: Supplements Packed with Nutrients

Add nutrient-rich leafy greens (which wilt quickly in the heat) to your stir-fries. Discover how adding greens to your stir-fries can improve their nutritional density by adding vitamins and minerals, such as bok choy and Swiss chard, in addition to spinach and kale.

Flavor Bombs and Aromatics: Instant Potency

Use flavor bombs and aromatics to give your stir-fries depth and quick impact. Learn how to add flavorful and savory ingredients to your nutrient-dense stir-fries, such as minced garlic, ginger, chili flakes, and soy sauce.

Quick Marinades and Sauces: Time-Saving Upgrades

Add flavorful and time-saving sauces and marinades to your stir-fries to make them even better. Discover how adding sauces and marinades, such as teriyaki and hoisin, to your nutrient-dense stir-fries may give a saucy and flavorful touch.

Seeds and Nuts: Crispy Ends

Nuts and seeds add a crunchy texture to your stir-fries. Find out how adding sesame seeds, cashews, peanuts, and almonds to your nutrient-dense stir-fries not only adds a pleasant crunch, but also adds healthy fats and proteins.

Easy Stir-Fry Combinations: Tasty Adjustments

Discover a range of rapid stir-fry combinations that may be customized to suit a variety of palates. Find a variety of nutrient-dense recipes that make stir-frying a fun and effective activity, from traditional tofu and vegetable stir-fries to hot peanut noodle varieties.

Hot Cooking Advice: Getting the Hang of the Wok

Gain mastery over the skill of cooking at high temperatures by learning how to use a wok. Discover how to use high heat to make quick, nutrient-dense stir fries, from getting the ideal sear on tofu to keeping veggies crisp.

Stir-Fry Dinner Prep: Effective Scheduling

Prepare your stir-fry meals in an efficient manner for hectic days. Find time-saving tips that turn nutrient-dense stir-fries into a practical option for quick and filling dinners, like pre-cutting veggies and marinating proteins.

Recipes to Satisfy Any Desire

Take a culinary adventure with these assortment of stir-fry dishes that are sure to satisfy any desire. Find a repertory of nutrient-dense stir-fries that make plant-powered cooking enjoyable and effective, from quick weeknight meals to inventive weekend ventures.

You will appreciate the speed and nutritional density of meals made with the skill of stir-frying, as well as the delight of colorful and savory bowls that support your vegan athletic lifestyle. Now is the perfect moment to mix, sizzle, and savor the nutrient-dense delight of plant-based stir fries.

Chapter 6: Snacks and Energy Boosters

Make Your Own Energy Bars

Improve your munching skills with these healthy, homemade energy bars. We'll explore the process of creating nutrient-dense bars in this chapter that will fuel your busy lifestyle while also satisfying your cravings. These baked energy bars range from easy no-bake recipes to inventive flavor combinations, celebrating healthy ingredients and delectable treats.

Alchemy of the Energy Bar: Creating Wholesome Goodness

Take on the art of creating homemade energy bars that are the ideal ratio of enjoyment to nourishment. Learn how to blend healthful ingredients to make bars that satisfy your palate and nourish your body.

Nutrient-Rich Base: The Energy Bar Foundation

Make a nutrient-rich bass for your energy bars, which will serve as the basis for these mouthwatering confections. Discover how these components—which range from seeds and dried fruits to nuts and rolled oats—provide a well-balanced combination of fiber, good fats, and vital nutrients.

Natural Sugar Substitutes: A Touch of Sugar

Us natural sweeteners to improve the flavor profile of your energy bars and add a hint of sweetness. Learn how various sweeteners, such as dates, maple syrup, agave nectar, and honey substitutes, add natural sugars without compromising the nutritional value of the food as a whole.

Protein Power: Increasing Fullness

Add some protein-rich ingredients to your energy bars to increase their satiety. Discover how various protein sources, which range from nut butters and plant-based protein powders to seeds like hemp and chia, can improve the durability of your homemade energy bars.

Tasty Add-Ins: Ingenious Upgrades

Use inventive additions to your energy bars to enhance their flavor profile and add excitement to each mouthful. Learn how these additions, which range from chocolate chips and coconut flakes to dried berries and spices, add texture and a pop of flavor.

Adhesive Agents: Guaranteeing Uniformity

Use binding agents to keep everything together and guarantee the coherence of your energy bars. Discover how these foods, which range from nut butters and date paste to mashed bananas and applesauce, make the ideal binding for your nutrient-dense recipes.

No-Bake Happiness: Easy Preparation

Discover the joy of making no-bake energy bars, while preparation yields great results. Find out how the lack of heat makes the entire process—from mixing and pressing to chilling—quick and simple.

Baked Delights: Crunch and Crinkle Textures

Discover baked energy bar recipes that provide a delicious blend of crunchy and chewy textures. Learn how baking gives your homemade energy bars a new depth, ranging from granola-like bars to soft and cakey types.

Tailored Recipes: Customized to Your Preferences

Adapt your energy bar recipes to your dietary requirements and personal tastes. You may tailor your snacking experience by adding new flavor combinations and modifying the sweetness levels of your DIY energy bars.

Portioning and Storing: Convenient Snack-Ready

Use appropriate portioning and storage strategies to guarantee snack-ready convenience. Learn how to turn your home-made energy bars into a handy and portable snack, from slicing them into the appropriate portions to keeping them in airtight containers or wrapping them for convenience of consumption on the spot.

Various Energy Bars: A Tasty Combination

Discover a tasty range of energy bar variants made to satisfy a variety of desires and tastes. Find a variety of recipes that transform homemade energy bars from traditional oat and nut bars to unique tropical and matcha-infused concoctions. These recipes make making energy bars at home a healthy and entertaining pastime.

Nut-Free and Ideal for Those with Allergies

If someone has dietary constraints, think about choosing nut-free and allergy-friendly products. Discover dishes that satisfy a variety of dietary restrictions and offer delectable substitutes for a broad spectrum of tastes, from seed-based snacks to oat-centric confections.

You'll discover that making your own energy bars is not only a fun and nourishing hobby, but it also allows you to create snacks that are ideal for your busy lifestyle. It's time to combine, press, and relish the healthful pleasure of homemade energy bars to support your transition to a vegan diet.

Nut mixtures with Roasted Chickpeas

Roasted chickpeas and nut mixes will add a crispy joy to your snacking. This will cover the art of making tasty, high-protein snacks that will fulfill your desires and give you a quick energy boost. These roasted masterpieces, which range from spicy spice blends to sweet and savory nut combinations, are a celebration of flavor, texture, and healthful deliciousness.

Snack Symphony: Crunchiness from Roasting

Come and join us for a munching symphony with roasted chickpeas and nut mixtures. Learn how to balance flavors, textures, and nutrients to make snacks that will satisfy your hunger and provide you with the energy you need.

Crunch of Chickpeas: The Roasted Wonder

Discover the wonder of roasted chickpeas as they turn from tender legumes into deliciously crunchy bites. Discover how different seasonings turn the plain chickpea into a snack-worthy pleasure with savory, spicy, and sweet versions.

Nut Mix Medley: Healthy, Protein-Packed

Mix a variety of nuts to create a protein-rich mix that gives your munchies a deep, satisfying crunch. Find out about the nutritional advantages of various nuts and how they go well with roasted chickpeas in your mixes, such as cashews, pistachios, and walnuts.

Flavorful Infusions with Savory Spice Blends

Infuse savory spice blends into your roasted chickpeas and nut combinations. Discover how these spices, which range from garlic and rosemary to smoky paprika and cumin, give your treats depth and complexity while balancing their flavors.

Nut-Crusted Harmony of Sweet and Salty

Achieve the ideal harmony between sweet and salty by utilizing nut combinations that entice your palate. Find out how adding a little sweetness to your roasted chickpeas and nut mixtures amplifies their overall decadence, from honey-roasted almonds to maple-glazed pecans.

Personalized Bundles: Adapting to Your Preferences

Adjust the nut mixtures and roasted chickpeas to your own personal preferences. Make your snacking experience unique and fulfilling by learning how to customize your snacks, from varying the amount of spice to trying out different nut combinations.

Herb-Infused Delight: Vibrant and New

Bring the flavor and fresh herbs to your munchies. Discover how adding herbs to your roasted chickpeas and nut mixes, such as thyme, oregano, dill, and basil, may infuse them with flavor and produce a delightfully fragrant and revitalizing experience.

Dried Fruit Supplements: Sweet and Crisp Treats

To your nuts mixes with dried fruits and roasted chickpeas, add some sweet and chewy treats. Find out how the fruity additions—from raisins and figs to cranberries and apricots—make a delightful counterpoint to the crisp texture of your snacks.

Spicy and Smoky Infusions: Vibrant Tastes

Use smoky and spicy infusions to infuse your roasted products with robust tastes. Discover how these bold and spice ingredients, which range from chipotle-lime almonds to sriracha-roasted chickpeas, enhance your snacks and leave a lasting imprint on your palate.

Portioning and Packaging: Convenient Snack-Ready

Use appropriate portioning and packaging strategies to guarantee snack-ready convenience. Learn how to make your snacks convenient to eat on-the-go, from utilizing resealable containers to storing your roasted chickpeas and nut mixtures in individual servings.

Festive Flavors of Seasonal Roasted Delights

Add festive and seasonal touches to your roasted chickpeas and nut mixes to calibrate the changing of the seasons. Discover how seasonal flavors add a little happiness to your snacking experience, from fruity pistachios in the summer to almonds flavored with pumpkin spice in the fall.

Recipes to Satisfy Any Desire

With a variety of roasted chickpeas and nut mix dishes to satisfy any craving, you may embark on a culinary adventure. Discover a variety of foods that can help you include roasted goodness into your vegan athlete lifestyle, from traditional smokey almonds to unique curry-spiced chickpeas.

You'll enjoy fulfilling snacks and the satisfaction of creating delectable, nutrient-dense bytes as you relish the crunchy delight of roasted chickpeas and nut mixtures. It's time to cook, combine, and savor the healthful goodness of snacks to support your athletic endeavors as a vegan.

Ideas for Fresh Fruit Snacking

In this chapter devoted to healthy and refreshing snacking, natural sweetness and vivid tastes of fresh fruits captivate your taste. Fresh fruit snacks are a celebration of nature's sweetness, from straightforward pairings to inventive combinations that not only satisfy your sweets but also provide your body with vital vitamins and minerals.

Sweet Symphony: The Candy Medley of Nature

Take in the natural sweetness and juiciness of fresh fruits as they take center stage in a fruity symphony. With nature's sweets, an array of hues, textures, and flavors that please and nourish your palate, you may learn the art of munching.

Fruit Bowls for One Serve: Simple Elegance

Single-serve fruit bowls that showcase the beauty of individual fruits and easy way to experience elegance. Discover how straightforward presentations, which range from cubed watermelon and pineapple to sliced strawberries and kiwis, enhance the pleasure and aesthetic appeal of snacking.

Layers of Happiness with Berry Bliss Parfaits

Berry bliss parfaits, which highlight the vivid colors and tastes of berries, are a delicious way to stack layers of goodness. Learn how these antioxidant-rich beauties, which range from strawberries to raspberries to blueberries, bring a burst of freshness to your snacking arsenal.

Citrus Feelings: Invigorating and Spicy

Savor zesty, revitalizing citrus flavors that tantalize your taste buds. Discover how the acidity of citrus fruits makes for a vibrant and energizing snack experience, with everything from chunks of luscious oranges and grapefruits to tart slices of kiwi and lime.

Tropical Fruit Heaven: Unique Treats

Take a trip to a tropical fruit paradise filled with delicious exotic treats to infuse your daily snacking routine with a hint of the tropics. Learn how tropical fruits, which range from chunks of mango and pineapple to coconut and papaya, lend a hint of escapism to your fresh fruit snacks.

Fruit Kabobs and Skewers: Delicious and Transportable

Fruit skewers and kabobs, which transform fresh fruits into bite-sized treats, add fun and portability to snacking. Discover how these imaginative displays, such as themed kabobs and rainbow fruit skewers, make snacking engaging and entertaining.

Rich and Nutritious Yogurt and Fruit Parfaits

Make healthy parfaits by combining the freshness of fruits with the creamy texture of yogurt. Find out how these yogurt parfaits, which range from coconut yogurt with layers of tropical fruit to Greek yogurt with honey-drizzled berries, offer a filling and high-protein snack alternative.

Fruit Dips with Nut Butter: Rich Combinations

Enjoy your fresh fruit munching to the fullest with delicious nut butter and fruit dip combinations. Discover how the creamy richness of nut butters gives your fruit snacks a pleasant twist, from almond butter with apple slices to chocolate-hazelnut dip with banana chunks.

Fruit Pops from Frozen: Chilled and revitalizing

Frozen fruit pops, which transform fresh fruits into frosty sweets, are a pleasant and delicious way to beat the heat. Find out how freezing fresh fruit results in a delicious and hydrating eating experience with everything from watermelon and mint popsicles to berry-infused ice pops.

Sweet and Spicy Fruit Salsa with Cinnamon Chips

Discover how cinnamon chips and fruit salsa combine to create a spicy and sweet mix that gives your usual snacking a fun twist. Learn how this creative mix produces a flavor-packed experience in anything from sliced mango and pineapple salsa to apple crisps coated with cinnamon.

Herbal Infusion Fruit Salad: Gourmet Style

Herb-infused fruit salads will add a touch of culinary flair to your fresh fruit munching. Discover how adding herbs to your fruit snacks enhances their flavor profile and gives them a sophisticated touch. Examples of such combinations include mint-infused melon mixtures and strawberry salads with basil kisses.

Season-Perfect Recipes

With a variety of fresh fruit snack recipes that can be made for any season, go on a seasonal adventure. Explore a variety of snacks that capture the flavor of each season on your tongue, from sweet watermelon concoctions in the summer to zesty treats in the winter.

Enjoying the healthy and energizing snack ideas with fresh fruits will make you feel good about feeding your body with nature's candy in addition to tasting delectable delicacies. Now is the perfect moment to cut, dice, and savor the deliciousness of fresh fruit snacks to support your vegan athletic lifestyle.

Chapter 7: Recovery Smoothies and Drinks

Smoothies with Protein After Exercise

Protein smoothies are a great way to replenish energy and revitalize your body after working out. This chapter will address the art of making tasty, nutrient-dense smoothies that are a refreshing and hydrating treat after a strenuous workout in addition to supporting muscle recovery. These protein smoothies are a celebration of taste and fitness, including everything from traditional combos to creative flavors.

Smoothie Recovery: Nutritious Following the Sweat

After working up a sweat, treat yourself to a smoothie resurrection, where the deliciousness of protein and nutrients come together in a reviving blend. Learn how to make protein smoothies that will satisfy your cravings and replenish your body after a workout.

A Base Packed with Protein: The Foundation for Muscle Repair

Create a basis for your smoothies that is high in protein to aid with muscle regeneration. Discover how various foods—from Greek yogurt and almond butter to silken tofu and plant-based protein powders—contribute vital amino acids to aid in the recuperation process following a workout.

Berry Blast: A Vitamin-Rich Drink

Berries provide a burst of flavor and antioxidants for a refreshing drink. Learn how these nutrient-dense berries, which range from raspberries and blackberries to blueberries and strawberries, not only bring sweetness but also help to reduce inflammation after exercise.

Tropical Heaven: Refreshing and Invigorating

Smoothies are a great way to hydrate and energize oneself while taking a trip to a tropical paradise. Discover how the tropical fruits in these smoothies—from kiwi and coconut water to pineapple and mango—provide a cool hit of taste and natural electrolytes.

Nutrient-Dense Greens: A Green Powerhouse

Add vitamin and mineral-rich, nutrient-dense greens to your smoothies after a workout. Learn how to incorporate leafy vegetables like spinach, kale, cucumber, and celery into your blends to provide color and antioxidants.

Creamy Nut Treats: Good Fats for Fullness

Nut-based healthy fats will improve creaminess and increase satiety in your smoothies. Discover how nutty ingredients, such as almond butter, cashews, chia seeds, and flaxseeds, contribute vital omega-3 fatty acids and add richness to food.

Banana Happiness: Innate Sugar and Potassium

Smoothies that highlight the inherent sweetness and potassium-rich qualities of bananas will make you feel like you're in banana nirvana. Find out how this adaptable fruit gives your post-workout blends a creamy texture and natural sweetness, whether you use it in traditional peanut butter and banana combos or in creative creations with dates.

Aloe Vera and Coconut Water for Hydration Boost

Use aloe vera and coconut water to your post-workout smoothies to increase the amount of hydration. Examine the ways that the calming effects of aloe vera and the electrolytes in coconut water aid in rehydration and recuperation following strenuous activity.

Chocolate Overindulgence: Rich Recuperation

Smoothies with chocolate added for a delightful post-workout recovery. Learn how the rich and velvety flavors of chocolate can transform your smoothies into a feast for your taste buds with everything from chocolate protein powders and cacao nibs to chocolate almond milk and hazelnut spread.

Coffee Infusions: Energizing Drinks

Smoothies containing coffee as an ingredient might provide your post-workout routine a caffeine boost. Discover how adding coffee to your blends can improve their flavor profile and offer an extra energy boost, from cold brew and espresso to protein powders flavored with coffee.

Ginger and Turmeric as Healing Elixirs

Use ginger and turmeric's anti-inflammatory properties to make healing concoctions. Learn how these fragrant and restorative spices aid in the recuperation process following a workout, from blends laced with ginger to golden smoothies seasoned with turmeric.

Recipes to Help You on Your Fitness Path

With a variety of post-workout protein smoothie recipes that are tailored to each fitness journey, start a tasty adventure. Discover a variety of smoothies that transform the post-workout ritual into a tasty and nutritious experience, ranging from muscle-building blinds to revitalizing recovery recipes.

Electrolyte drinks that hydrate

Electrolyte drinks are a great way to stay hydrated while replenishing your electrolytes. This chapter will cover the craft of making refreshing drinks that replenish vital minerals lost during exercise in addition to keeping you well-hydrated. These electrolyte beverages, which range from tasty blends to natural infusions, are a celebration of taste and hydration.

Electrolyte Resupply: The Crucial Hydration

Explore the realm of electrolyte replacement, where staying hydrated becomes crucial for leading an active lifestyle. Learn how to make delicious, nutrient-rich beverages that go beyond water to keep you hydrated and feeling energi sed.

DIY Sports Drink Foundation: Personalized Hydration

Make a hydration foundation that you can customize for your electrolyte drinks. Discover how these basic ingredients can be used to create electrolyte drinks that are customized to your preferences and dietary requirements, ranging from coconut water and citrus juices to herbal teas and natural sweeteners.

Vitamin C Boost: Citrus Burst

Have an explosion of citrus flavor with vitamin C-enriched electrolyte drinks. Learn how the zesty acidity of citrus fruits improves the refreshing quality of your hydrating beverages, from lemon and lime-infused waters to orange and grapefruit cocktails.

Coconut Oasis: A Natural Supplement for Electrolytes

With the hydrating properties of coconut water, turn your electrolyte drinks into a tropical paradise. Learn how this natural elixir replaces electrolytes and gives your beverages a tropical touch. Try it straight or blended with pineapple or watermelon.

Berries Infusions: A Vitamin-Rich Drink

Bring the berries and their antioxidant content to your electrolyte drinks. From strawberry and blackberry blends to waters flavored with blueberries and raspberries, see how these colorful fruits not only improve flavor but also add vital vitamins that promote general health.

Herbal Hydration: A Touch of Class

Use botanical components to inject elegance and elevate your electrolyte drinks. Discover how these herbs, which range from mint and basil to rosemary and thyme, can enhance the taste, scent, and even health benefits of your hydration drinks.

Wave of Watermelon: Refreshing and Nourishing

Drink electrolyte beverages, which are cooling and hydrating, to ride the watermelon wave. Find out how the high water content and inherent sweetness of watermelon make it a delicious option for your daily hydration regimen, whether you're drinking pure watermelon juice or blending it with cucumber.

Ginger Zing: Energizing the Stomach

Ginger's energizing flavor can give your electrolyte drinks a boost. Learn about the possible digestive and anti-inflammatory properties of this spicy root by trying out recipes like ginger-infused lemonades or elixirs combining ginger and turmeric.

Salted Orange Peel: Sodium Equilibrium

To guarantee proper sodium levels, add a zesty, salty edge to your electrolyte drinks. Learn how sodium is essential for keeping hydrated and avoiding dehydration with everything from a sprinkling of sea salt in lemon water to homemade sports drinks with a sodium boost.

Electrolyte Treats: Frozen Hydration Popsicles

Hydration popsicles are a great way to turn electrolyte liquids into frozen sweets. Discover how these cool treats make staying hydrated enjoyable and delectable, from freezing your favorite electrolyte blends into popsicle molds to adding bits of fruit for texture.

Green Tea Elixir: Powerful Antioxidant

Put some green tea's potent antioxidants in your electrolyte drinks. Explore the various combinations of green tea and honey and citrus blinds to see how this traditional drink enhances flavor and may have health advantages.

Recipes for Any Need for Hydration

With a variety of electrolyte drink recipes to suit all hydration requirements, set out on a tasty adventure. Discover a variety of beverages that make staying hydrated a tasty and healthful habit, from post-workout refreshment to summer coolers and immune-boosting elixirs.

You'll not only satisfy your thirst as you navigate the world of hydrating electrolyte drinks, but you'll also feel good about making drinks that complement your active and health-conscious lifestyle. Now is the moment to pour, take a sip, and enjoy the deliciously hydrating drinks that will leave you feeling rejuvenated and energi sed.

Superfood Elixirs in Green

Green superfood elixirs have the nutritious capacity to elevate your wellness journey. This chapter will cover the skill of making nutrient-rich, energizing elixirs that will not only enhances your general health but also add a tasty and colorful touch to your everyday routine. These recipes, which range from immune-boosting to detoxifying blends, are a celebration of flavor and vibrancy in green drinks.

Superfood Alchemy: Vitality's Elixir

Sét out on a voyage of superfood alchemy, where the vivid colors and nutrient-dense deliciousness of greens combine to create a revitalizing elixir. Learn how to make nourishing green superfood elixirs that awaken your senses and replenish your body.

Green Elixir Base: Foundations Rich in Nutrients

Build a nutrient-rich base for your green drinks. Discover how these superfoods—which range from wheatgrass and chlorella to leafy greens and spirulina—offer a wealth of vitamins, minerals, and antioxidants that promote general wellbeing.

Detoxifying Concoctions: Purifying Green Energy

Detoxifying green elixirs can help your body get clean and refreshed. Learn how these elixirs, which range from kale and cucumber blends to parsley and lemon infusions, can create a healthy and regenerated system by eliminating pollutants.

Entire Armor for Health: Green Immunity Boosters

Green elixirs are health-protective armor that help strengthen your immune system. Explore how the antioxidant-rich components enhance immune system function and general resilience in everything from spinach and ginger combinations to green tea and kiwi blends.

Energizing Blends: Eco-Friendly Energy for Exercise

Energize your body with green elixirs to give it the duel it needs. Try smoothies with matcha and banana or drinks with spinach and pineapple to see how the balance of natural sugars and greens can support your busy lifestyle.

Antioxidant Chorus: Bright Skin Toners

Encourage glowing skin with green drinks that create a symphony of antioxidants. Discover how these elixirs, which range from cucumber and mint drinks to avocado and kale mixtures, support healthy skin by battling oxidative stress and fostering a natural shine.

Gut-Friendly Greens: Digestive Elixirs

Boost digestive health with green elixirs that are beneficial to the gut. Learn how these elixirs improve digestion, lessen bloating, and foster a healthy gut environment with everything from probiotic-rich kefir and spinach mixes to mint and fennel infusions.

Green Quenchers: Hydration Elixirs

Drink more than just water to quench your thirst with hydrating green drinks. Discover how these drinks, which range from cucumber and aloe vera to coconut water and kale mixtures, not only hydrate but also include vital nutrients to keep you feeling reenergized.

Cognitive Clarity: Brain-Boosting Elixirs

Use brain-healthy green elixirs to improve cognitive clarity. Learn how these concoctions, which range from avocado and green tea mixes to smoothies with blueberries and spinach, offer a mix of nutrients and antioxidants that support mental clarity and alertness.

Calming Recipes: Stress-Relieving Mixtures

Calming green elixirs encourage relaxation and relieve tension. Discover how these elixirs, which range from cucumber beverages with lavender infusion to combinations of chamomile and kale, promote calmness and wellbeing.

Harmony of Sweet and Savory Tastes: Delightful Nuance

Savory and sweet green elixirs will provide you with a complex flavor experience. Discover how the blending of various flavors results in a delightful and fulfilling elixir experience, from beet and kale juices with a hint of apple sweetness to spinach and avocado smoothies with a tinge of lime.

Recipes for Optimal Daily Health

Set off on a quest for daily vitality with a variety of green superfood elixir recipes tailored to meet different requirements. Discover a variety of concoctions that will turn eating more greens into a delightful and healthy habit, from morning pick-me-ups to nighttime relaxation mixes.

You will not only provide your body with vital nutrients as you navigate the world of green superfood elixirs, but you will also get a kick out of creating drinks that promote your general health. It's time to mix, drink, and savor the energy of elixirs that support you on your path to a more energetic and healthy existence.

Chapter 8: Meal Planning and Prep Tips

7-day vegan meal plans for athletes

A range of high-protein plant-based foods, including tofu, tempeh, beans, lentils, quinoa, nuts, seeds, and soy products, are included in our 7-day vegan athletes meal plans.

Other essential minerals for vegan athletes included in these foods are iron, zinc, calcium, iodine, and vitamin B12.

We have also included various omega-3 fatty acid sources, like hemp seeds, walnuts, chia seeds, and flaxseeds. These fats help to lower inflammation, enhance cardiovascular health, and improve cognitive function.

Day 1:

- **Blueberry, Banana smoothie bowl for breakfast**

Plant milk, frozen banana, frozen blueberries, vegan protein powder, and ground flaxseed combine to create a creamy smoothie. Add sliced banana, almonds, chia seeds, granola, and fresh blueberries over top.

- **Snack: Peanut butter on an apple**

Cut an apple into thin slices, apply peanut butter, and then top with flaxseed.

- **Brown rice and tofu veggie stir-fry for lunch**

A tasty stir-fry consisting of crispy tofu cubes tossed in a sauce that is both sweet and spicy. Accompany with cooked brown rice and sauteed broccoli.

- **Trail mix snack:** a chewy and crunchy combination of chunks of dark chocolate, dried cranberries, and raw almonds.
- **Dinner is pasta with healthy grains and lentil bolognese.**

Made with cooked lentils simmered in a tomato sauce with herbs and spices, this dish is filling and substantial. Garnish with vegan parmesan cheese or nutritional yeast and serve over spaghetti.

Day 2:

- **Oatmeal with peanut butter and banana for breakfast**

Almond butter, mashed banana, rolled oats, and water (or plant milk) are combined to make warm or overnight oatmeal. Add sliced berries, almonds, and chia seeds over top.

- **Snack: Carrot sticks with hummus**

A tasty and creamy dip consisting of chickpeas, tahini, lemon juice, garlic, and salt. Accompany with whole grain crackers, veggie sticks, or carrot sticks.

- **Lunch would be roasted chickpeas and quinoa salad.**

Cooked quinoa, chopped kale, cherry tomatoes, cucumber, avocado, olives, and dressing combine to make a light and satisfying salad. Add roasted chickpeas that have been seasoned with paprika, salt, and pepper on top.

- **Chocolate protein shake for a snack**

Made with plant milk, frozen banana, ice, vegan chocolate protein powder, and cocoa powder, this smoothie is rich and filling.

- **Dinner is sweet potato fries and tempeh veggie burgers.**

A tasty and wholesome burger consisting of crumbled tempeh, onion, carrot, garlic, soy sauce, and oats. Arrange your preferred toppings on top of whole-wheat buns. Serve alongside some sweet potato fries that have been seasoned with paprika, salt, and pepper.

Day 3:

- **Whole grain bread and tofu scramble for breakfast**

A flavorful, high-protein scramble cooked with nutritional yeast, onion, garlic, turmeric, and crumbled tofu, seasoned with salt and pepper. cooked till fluffy and golden. Served with vegan butter (or jam) and whole-wheat bread.

- **Granola bars as a snack**

Made with oats, almonds, seeds, peanut butter, dried fruit, maple syrup, and salt, this bar is chewy and crispy. Baked or left undone until solid, then sliced into bars.

- **Lunch is a salsa-topped black bean tortilla.**

Made on a whole-wheat tortilla and packed with black beans, rice, corn, lettuce, tomato, avocado, and vegan cheese (or nutritional yeast), this burrito is flavorful and spicy. Combine fresh tomato salsa with freshly toasted toast and fold.

- **Snack: Berries and yogurt**

a tart and creamy snack made with frozen or fresh berries and vegan yogurt (such as soy or coconut yogurt). Add some nuts, seeds, and granola on top.

- **Dinner is naan bread and vegetable curry.**

A rich, aromatic curry cooked with coconut milk. Add the cilantro, spinach, chickpeas, and cauliflower and simmer. Serve with rice or naan bread.

Day 4

- **Chia pudding with mango for breakfast**

A silky and velvet pudding prepared by soaking chia seeds in plant milk for a whole night in the refrigerator. Add some vanilla extract and maple syrup and stir. Add some shredded coconut and mango chunks, either frozen or fresh, on top.

- **Edamame with sea salt for a snack**

A straightforward and filling snack consisting of steamed or boiled edamame pods seasoned with sea salt. Remove the beans from the pods to peel and consume.

- **Lunch would be roasted tempeh and kale salad.**

Chopped kale is mixed with olive oil, nutritional yeast, and lemon juice to create a crunchy and filling salad. Add roasted tempeh cubes and toss. Sunflower seeds and dehydrated cranberries should be added.

- **Munchies made with banana bread**

Made with whole-wheat flour, flax eggs, and mashed ripe bananas, this muffin is moist and fluffy. Add chocolate chips and some chopped walnuts. Place in a muffin tray and bake until done and golden.

- **Dinner is bread and vegetable soup.**

Made with vegetable broth, carrot, celery, potato, corn, green beans, peas, and barley, this soup is hearty and warming. Simmer until fragrant and tender. served with vegan butter (or jam), if desired, and whole-wheat toast.

Day 5:

- **Avocado toast with scrambled tofu for breakfast**

Avocado toast with scrambled tofu for breakfast is a filling and tasty whole-wheat bread toast topped with mashed avocado. Add crushed tofu and nutritional yeast to make scrambled tofu on top. Present alongside a portion of raw berries.

- **Snack: Pear and oatmeal cookie**

Made with oats, whole-wheat flour, vegan butter, flax egg, and dried sour cherries, this cookie is chewy and incredibly tasty. Savor it alongside a crisp apple or pear.

- **Hummus and veggie wrap for lunch**

A delicious and substantial wrap made with a whole-wheat tortilla smeared with hummus and stuffed with carrot, bell pepper, lettuce, tomato, cucumber, and olives along with tempeh. chopped into bite-sized pieces or rolled and then cut in half.

- **Snack: Yogurt-topped fruit salad**

A light and sweet salad consisting of vegan yogurt (such as soy or coconut yogurt) and diced fresh fruit. topped with chia seeds and some shredded coconut.

- **Dinner is noodles and mushroom stroganoff.**

Sliced mushrooms are sautéed with onion, garlic, salt, pepper, and paprika to create a creamy and flavorful dish. To thicken the sauce, stir in some plant milk or vegan sour cream. Server with a crisp green salad and cooked noodles or rice.

Day 6:

- **Yogurt and granola with berries for breakfast**

Granola and vegan yogurt combine to make a crunchy and creamy breakfast. topped with berries, either frozen or fresh, and a variety of nuts and seeds, including sunflower, walnut, and almond seeds.

- **Popcorn with nutritional yeast for a snack**

A straightforward and filling snack consisting of popping popcorn kernels in a pot with oil and adding nutritional yeast (or salt) for a cheese taste.

- **Lunch is fries and a burger.**

Made with a vegetarian burger patty and a whole-wheat bun, this burger is tasty and healthy. Add lettuce, tomato, onion, and your preferred sauces on top. Accompany potato wedges roasted in the oven and seasoned with salt, pepper, and oil.

- **Chocolate chip cookies as a snack**

Made with whole-wheat flour, chocolate chips, vanilla essence, vegan butter, and flax egg, these cookies are soft and chewy.

- **Dinner is lasagna with veggies.**

This recipe is cheesy and comforting, consisting of layers of vegan ricotta cheese (made with tofu, lemon juice, and nutritional yeast), vegan mozzarella cheese, vegan parmesan cheese, and tomato sauce over lasagna noodles.

Day 7:

- **Berries and maple syrup on pancakes for breakfast**

A light and delectable breakfast consisting of plant milk (almond or soy), vegan butter, vanilla essence, and whole-wheat flour. Top with frozen or fresh berries and extra maple syrup.

- **Almonds roasted for a snack**

Raw almonds roasted in the oven with oil, salt, pepper, rosemary, and thyme create a crisp and flavorful snack.

- **Lunch would be soy-sauced vegetable sushi.**

A delicious and entertaining sushi rice meal. Arrange on a nori seaweed sheet, then add sliced bell pepper, avocado, cucumber, and carrot on top. Cut into pieces after rolling. Serve with ginger, wasabi, and soy sauce (or tamari).

- **Snack: Nut balls and dates**

A chewy and sweet snack consisting of almonds, cocoa powder, salt, vanilla extract, and pitted dates. Blend or process in a food processor until smooth and sticky. Shape into spheres and cover with grated coconut.

- **Dinner is vegetable and bean. Chili and cornbread**

Using onion, garlic, cumin, chili powder, salt, pepper, and whatever additional flavors you like, this recipe is meaty and spicy. Cook alongside green beans, corn, kidney beans, smashed tomatoes, and black beans. Accompany with vegan sour cream and cornbread.

Techniques for Freezing and Batch Cooking for Busy Vegan Athletes

These batch cooking and freezing techniques combine efficiency and nutrition to make meal preparation easier for busy vegan athletes. You can fill your freezer with healthy, ready-to-eat meals by setting aside a few hours to cook. This will guarantee that you always have nourishing options available, even on the busiest days.

Fundamentals of Batch Cooking:

1. **Laying the groundwork Ingredient Preparation:**
   - Lettuces, cereals, and veggies be washed, chopped, and portioned ahead of time.

To save time over the week, prepare staple grains like lentils, brown rice, and quinoa in advance.

2. **Multi-Tasking Magic:** Cook different parts of meals at the same time by using your oven and multiple burners.
   - Roast veggies or saute protein sources while the grains are simmering.

3. **Crafty Sauce Creation:** Construct adaptable sauces and dressings that complement a wide range of foods.
   - To make thawing and using sauces easier, portion them into ice cube trays.

Methods of Freezing: Optimizing Freshness

1. **Cooling Procedures:** To preserve texture, let cooked ingredients cool fully before freezing.
   - For faster cooling, lay goods out on trays or shallow containers.

2. **Portion control:** To be flexible, freeze meals in portions that are appropriate for an individual or a family.

- To freeze little amounts of condiments, herbs, or sauces, use silicone molds.

3. **Air-Tight Packaging:** To reduce freezer burn, firmly wrap products in plastic wrap or place them in vacuum-sealed containers.

- For tracking, mark containers with the preparation date.
- Invest in glass or plastic containers made specifically for use in freezers.
- In order to allow for food growth during freezing, leave a tiny opening at the top.

Recipes for Batch Cooking: Time-Reducing Pleasures

1. **One-Pot Wonders:** Make big batches of robust stews, soups, or chili for simple reheating.

- Individual portions can be frozen for easy and filling dinners.

2. **Baked Goodies:** Make a big batch of vegan enchiladas, lasagnas, or casseroles.

- For easy warming and portion control, slice before freezing. Protein Power

3. **Packs:** Use various marinades to batch-cook proteins such as seitan, tempeh, or tofu.
- Freeze in appropriate sizes for high-protein additions to different recipes.

4. **Grain Spree:** Prepare a ton of grains, such as barley, quinoa, and farro.
- Freeze in sections to use as a base for different recipes or as quick sides.

Tips for Thawing and Heating: Restoring Freshness

1. **Strategies for Thawing:**
- A day in advance, place frozen goods in the refrigerator to gradually defrost.
- For faster outcomes, use your microwave's defrost function.

2. **Perfect Reheating:** Use the cooktop to reheat soups and stews to a consistent temperature.
- Reheat casseroles or baked goods in the oven or toaster oven.

3. **Fresh Garnishes:** To add a taste explosion after reheating, add avocado, fresh herbs, or a squeeze of citrus.
- Add the raw toppings right before serving, keeping them separate.

Savvy Grocery Purchasing for Foods High in Nutrients

Make smart buying decisions that complement your vegan athlete lifestyle to up your shopping game. This will cover the art of strategic grocery shopping, which will help you fill your basket with nutrient-dense foods that will fuel your body to function at its best by helping you purposefully navigate the aisles.

1. Get Ready for Pre-Shopping:

- **Meal Planning:** Make a focused shopping list by planning your meals and snacks for the coming week.
- **Examine the pantry:** Make a list of everything you own to prevent having extra copies.

2. Shop the Periphery:

- **Fresh Vegetables:** In order to guarantee a range of nutrients, load up on colorful fruits and veggies.
- **Plant-Based Proteins:** Look for tofu, tempeh, lentils, and plant-based protein sources in the fresh or frozen area.

3. Whole Grains & Legumes:

- **Bulk Bin Section:** Purchasing in bulk will save you money on mainstays like quinoa, brown rice, lentils, and oats.
- **Diverse Grains:** For diversity, try out old grains like bulgur, farro, and barley.

4. Frozen Basics:

- **Greens and Berries:** Keep leafy greens on hand for easy cooking and freeze-dried berries for smoothies.
- **Frozen Vegetables:** For easy meal additions, make sure your frozen vegetable selection is diverse.

5. Non-Dairy Milk: Plant-Powered Dairy Alternatives Select from plant-based milks such as oat, soy, almond, or others.

- **Plant-Based Yogurt:** For extra health advantages, choose types enhanced with probiotics and vitamins.

6. Healthy Fats:

- **Avocado and Nuts:** To get healthy fats, add avocados and a range of nuts to your shopping basket.
- **Cooking Oils:** Use plant-based oils, such as olive oil, for dressings and cooking.

7. Smart Snacking:

- **Fresh Snacks:** For easy snacking, grab some chopped vegetables, fresh fruits, or preportioned hummus.
- **Nuts and Seeds:** To obtain a rapid energy boost, grab a variety of nuts and seeds.

8. Herbs and Spices:

- **Fresh Herbs:** Use fresh herbs like mint, cilantro, and parsley to accentuate flavors.
- **Spice Blends:** Try different spice mixtures to give your food more flavor without adding too much sodium.

9. Products Using Whole Ingredients:

- **Check Labels:** Select goods that include only whole-food ingredients.
- **Eat Less Processed Food:** Steer clear of meals and snacks that have a lot of additives.

10. Basics for Meal Prep:

- **Essential Containers:** Reusable containers are an investment for meal preparation.
- **Staples for Bulk Purchases:** Invest in bulk purchases of pantry essentials like grains, beans, and seeds to save money.

11. Making Sustainable and Ethical Decisions:

- **Regional Produce:** By selecting seasonal and local produce, you may lessen your carbon footprint and help local farmers.
- Choose brands that uphold ethical and sustainable standards.

12. Conscientious Budgeting:

- **Promotions and Rebates:** Benefit from discounts and sales when making large purchases.
- **Seasonal vegetables:** To get the best deals and freshest vegetables, buy seasonal produce.

The ability to shop for groceries wisely is one that comes with experience. Intentionally choosing nutrient-dense foods will help you live a healthier, more sustainable lifestyle in addition to maximizing your athletic performance. Cheers to your shopping!

Chapter 9: Vegan Supplements for Athletes

Recognizing Nutrient Shortfalls in a Vegan Diet for Athletes

Explore the subtleties of a vegan athlete's diet to learn about any possible dietary deficiencies. This chapter will cover the key nutrients, where to find them, and practical tips for maintaining a balanced, well-rounded diet that can help you succeed in your athletic pursuits.

1. **Protein:** Recognize that while plant-based sources of protein are sufficient, make sure to provide a range of amino acids to satisfy all necessary ones.

   Make strategic decisions by combining grains, seeds, and legumes to increase protein intake.

2. **Iron**: Recognize that non-heme iron derived from plants may be more difficult to absorb.

   Make strategic decisions by combining foods high in iron with sources of vitamin C to improve absorption. If required, take into account fortified foods and supplements.

3. **Calcium**: Recognize that while dairy is a common source of calcium, there are many plant-based substitutes available.

Make wise decisions by including fortified non dairy milk, tofu, leafy greens, and almonds in your diet.

4. **Vitamin B12:** Recognize that this vitamin, which is mostly found in animal products, is necessary for the metabolism of energy.

Using supplements or fortified meals can help you reach your B12 requirements.

5. **Omega-3 Fatty Acids:**

Knowledge: Although fish is a popular source, plant-based sources of ALA include flaxseeds and walnuts.

Strategic Decisions: For a well-rounded omega-3 diet, include flaxseeds, chia seeds, hemp seeds, and algae-based supplements.

6. **Vitamin D:** Recognize that while sunlight is a natural supply, there aren't many dietary sources.

Strategic Decisions: If exposure to sunshine is inadequate, take into account supplements, mushrooms, and fortified foods.

7. **Zinc:**

Knowledge: Zinc comes from plants, however phytates may prevent it from being absorbed.

Make strategic decisions by including foods high in zinc, such as nuts, seeds, and legumes. To boost bioavailability, think about soaking and sprouting.

8. **Iodine:** Recognize that while seaweed is a powerful source, plant meals vary in their iodine levels.

   Strategic Decisions: Incorporate seaweed into your diet and use iodized salt. If necessary, think about taking supplements.

9. **Understanding:** Known to be present in animal products, creatine aids in the generation of energy during strenuous exercise.

   Strategies: If you want to perform at your best in sports, think about taking creatine supplements.

10. **Carnosine:** Know that this protein, which is high in meat, possesses antioxidant qualities.

    Make wise decisions by emphasizing a diet high in beta-alanine, which is derived from plant sources and is a precursor to carnosine.

11. **Taurine: Knowledge:** Taurine, which is mostly present in animal products, is involved in cardiovascular health.

    Make decisions by concentrating on a plant-based diet that is well-balanced or by taking taurine supplements.

12.   **L-Carnitine:**

Knowledge: This amino acid, which is present in meat, helps in the metabolism of energy.

Strategic Decisions: Since lysine can be a precursor to L-carnitine, make sure you're getting enough of it from beans, quinoa, and tofu.

13.   **Choline:**

Knowledge: Rich in choline, which is crucial for liver function, are animal products.

Make strategic decisions by including plant sources such as broccoli, quinoa, and soy. If necessary, think about taking supplements.

For a vegan diet to maximize athletic performance, it is imperative to recognize and fill in dietary deficiencies. Making well-informed decisions and including a range of nutrient-dense foods will help you meet your nutritional requirements and achieve your overall fitness and health objectives.

Essential Vegan Supplements for Optimal Sports Results

Discover how vegan vitamins can improve your performance and promote general health. We'll look at key supplements in this chapter that are critical to filling up nutrient gaps and maximizing your athletic performance.

1. **Vitamin B12:**

  - **Function:** Essential for neurological function and energy metabolism.
  - **Source:** B12 pills or fortified meals.
  - **Benefits:** Enhanced energy and mental performance.

2. The role of omega-3 fatty acids is to reduce inflammation and support cardiovascular health.

  - **Source:** Hemp, chia, and flaxseed seeds; supplements containing algae oil.
  - **Advantages:** Improved joint health and recuperation.

3. **Vitamin D:** Immune system and bone health depend on it.

  - **Source:** Vitamin D pills, meals enriched with minerals, or sun exposure.
  - **Benefits:** Immune system support and stronger bones.

4. **Iron:**

  - **Function:** Essential for oxygen transportation and fatigue prevention.
  - **Source:** Iron-rich plant-based diets and supplements, if required.
  - **Advantages:** Enhanced stamina and vitality.

5. **Calcium:**

  - **Function:** Promotes the health of bones and muscles.

- **Source:** Tofu, calcium supplements, and fortified nondairy milk, if needed.
- **Benefits:** Ideal muscle function and strong bones.

6. **Zinc:** Immune system performance and wound healing depend on zinc.

- **Source:** Nuts, seeds, legumes, and, if needed, zinc supplements.
- **Advantages:** Better recuperation and immunological support.

7. **Creatine:**

- **Function:** Promotes the synthesis of energy during intense physical activity.
- Supplements containing creatine sourced non-animally.
- **Gains:** Increased power, strength, and muscle repair.

8. **Taurine:**

- **Function:** Promotes healthy heart and muscles.
- **Source:** Plant-based sources such as seaweed or supplements containing taurine.
- **Benefits** include improved cardiovascular health and maybe improved performance.

9. **L-carnitine:**

- **Function:** Aids in the movement of fats for energy.
- **Source:** Ensure appropriate lysine intake from plant sources.

- **Benefits:** May aid in recuperation and endurance.

10. **Choline:**

- **Function:** Essential for neurotransmitter and liver functioning.
- **Source:** Sources of plant-based choline, such as broccoli, quinoa, and soy.
- **Benefits:** Maximum liver health and mental clarity.

11. **Iodine:**

- **Function:** Critical to metabolism and thyroid function.
- Seaweed, iodized salt, and, if necessary, iodine supplements are the sources.
- **Benefits:** Thyroid health and regulated metabolism.

12. Exercise-related buffering of lactic acid is provided by beta-alanine, which serves as a precursor to carnosine.

- **Source:** Supplements containing carnosine and plant-based foods like lentils.
- **Advantages:** Lessened muscle fatigue and increased endurance.

13. **Supplements with Lysine:**

- **Function:** Essential for protein synthesis and a precursor to L-carnitine.
- **Source:** Foods high in lysine or supplements made from plants.

- **Advantages:** Promotes the synthesis of muscle proteins and enhances athletic performance.

Chapter 10: Success Stories

Indeed, success tales can provide a great deal of inspiration. Allow me to present a few to you:

1. Emily's Path to Olympic Success:

Meet Emily, a dedicated vegan runner who changed to a plant-based diet and lifestyle that improved both her physical and general health. A few years ago, Emily began running marathons, but she struggled with exhaustion and recuperation. She made the decision to go vegan because she was intrigued by the possible advantages of the diet.

Emily made a point of eating a wide range of fruits, vegetables, whole grains, and plant-based proteins as well as other nutrient-dense foods. To fill in any possible nutritional shortfalls, she purposefully included vitamins like iron, omega-3 fatty acids, and vitamin B12.

The outcomes were astounding. Emily found that she recovered from injuries more quickly in addition to having more energy. Her marathon times dropped dramatically, and she set new records in a number of races. Emily's experience is proof of the transformational potential of a plant-based diet that is well-balanced for sports achievement.

2. Jason's Muscle Gains Powered by Plants:

Devoted to weightlifting, Jason adopted a vegan lifestyle to refute the myth that plant-based diets are insufficient in protein to support muscular growth. He carefully prepared his meals, emphasizing a range of plant-based sources such as lentils, tofu, tempeh, and seitan, to guarantee a sufficient intake of protein.

Supplements like protein powder and creatine were also used by Jason to help him reach his muscle-building objectives. Jason's overall well-being and muscular mass were maintained along with faster recovery periods through consistent training and nutrition.

His success story dispelled myths about veganism and muscle growth while also encouraging other members of the fitness community to investigate plant-powered gains.

These success tales demonstrate the variety of ways people can achieve their fitness objectives and survive on a vegan diet. They highlight the significance of careful meal planning, nutrient-aware selections, and, occasionally, well-timed supplementation. Though every journey is different, these accounts show how adopting a plant-based lifestyle may lead to excellence.

CONCLUSION

To sum up, becoming a vegan athlete is an exciting and fulfilling journey that highlights the body's resiliency when fed a plant-based diet. This thorough book aims to empower and inspire readers with everything from comprehending the principles of a balanced vegan diet to discovering creative recipes and embracing strategic supplementation.

Keep these things in mind as you start your vegan athletic journey:

Nutritional Awareness: Pay attention to the nutrients you consume and make sure your diet is varied and well-rounded to suit your needs as an athlete.

Creative Cooking: Take use of the wide variety of plant-based products to make every me al a tasty and healthy affair.

Strategic Supplementation: To fill in dietary gaps and improve performance, take supplements when necessary.

Community and Support: Get involved in the lively vegan athlete community by exchanging ideas, knowledge, and inspiration.

Growth and Adaptation: Welcome the ongoing growth of your path, modifying your strategy in response to feedback from events and your body.

You will not only succeed as a vegan athlete but also add to the growing story of plant-powered success by developing a solid foundation of nutritional knowledge, experimenting with tasty and nutrient-dense recipes, and remaining involved in the community.

Remember that every step you take toward a more mindful and compassionate lifestyle is a step towards holistic well-being and athletic excellence, regardless of how experienced you are in the gym or if you are just beginning your fitness journey. Cheers to your success, health, and vigor as you embark on the thrilling journey of being a vegan athlete!

REVIEW PAGE

Dear Reader,

I hope this correspondence finds you well. I hope you've had fun perusing my most current, in-depth guide to vegan athleticism. I value your opinions and insights very much, so I would be very grateful if you could take a moment to let me know what you think.

Your comments will help me make my content better every time, and they will also help me create more useful and customized resources for you and other people who are interested in the vegan athlete lifestyle.

Would you kindly take a few minutes to discuss the following with me?

Which parts of the manual are most beneficial to you?

Are there any particular subjects that you would like to see more of?

Did you find the informational and engaging content?

Please feel free to add any more remarks or recommendations you may have.

I sincerely appreciate your time and advice. I sincerely appreciate your help in improving the value and enrichment of my work.

Warm regards,

Artem Zhdanov